Welcome to Smoothie World

Unlock EVERY Secret of Cooking

Through 500 AMAZING

Smoothie Recipes

(Unlock Cooking, Book 22)

Annie Kate

Contents

Introduction

***

"To keep the body in good health is a duty... otherwise we shall not be able to keep our mind strong and clear."

___Buddha__

No one can deny the importance of health in our lives. It's health, as Mahatma Gandhi said, that is the real wealth not pieces of gold and silver. A good health is not something you can buy, but a thing you can improve considerably with a few changes in your lifestyle. Notably, chasing a healthy life is a long-term commitment, not a flash-in-the-pan fad. However, thanks to smoothies, you can right now make today healthier than yesterday and pave the way for healthy living tomorrow, too.

Smoothie has been a favorite beverage in popularity recently. It's famous for various magical benefits including ***anti-inflammatory, antioxidant, heart health, weight loss, immune system***. It's really awesome, but what is smoothie exactly? What makes it so good?

A smoothie is a thick beverage made from blended raw fruits or vegetables with other ingredients such as water, ice, dairy products or sweeteners. Smoothie is best choice for your healthy lifestyle because it can extract every last drops of goodness from fruits and vegetables and then bring them naturally to your body. Only with a glass of fresh smoothie every morning can you receive a boost of ***mineral, vitamins, antioxidant, fiber*** and many ***other essential nutrients***. Not only does smoothie nourish your body in a quick and easy way but it also keeps your body fit and makes your skin more youthful day after day. The greatest thing of smoothie, in my opinion, is that it is suitable for everyone even for the busiest person, as it just takes you a matter of seconds to make. Let's cut, dice some of your favorite fruits and vegetable, then put all of them in a blender, add some fresh water press a button. And it's done. You have just made a delicious and nutritious for yourself. That's so simple, right?

We all know that everything has both sides: negative and positive. And smoothie, according to some recent researches, is not an exception. All smoothies are **NOT** created equal. Beside a lot of healthy kinds of smoothies, there are a number of kinds which cause harm to your health. They're the root of many health problems such as increasing **dryness, roughness, coldness, mobility and variability in the body/mind.** I can guarantee that information is correct and reliable, as I myself have ever got those problems because of consuming wrong smoothies. Therefore, in this book, before providing you with **500 smoothie recipes,** I'll give you enough essential information about pros and cons of smoothie. Right after reading some very first pages, you'll be able to discern between healthy and unhealthy smoothies with ease. Surely, you'll know the right way to gain all benefits of smoothie as well. Congratulate you on it!

I find myself really lucky because I can spend most of my time taking care of my family. Preparing nutritious meals for my husband and my children every single day and seeing them glad and healthy all the time is my biggest happiness. I really want to share that happiness with other people, especially with busy women who just have a little time but still want to guarantee healthy life for their families. It's the reason why I wrote this book "**Welcome to the world of smoothie**" includes some following chapters:

- *Chapter 1: Top 10 Benefits of Smoothies*
- *Chapter 2: Top 10 Tips for Better Smoothies*

500 AMAZING Smoothie Recipes, which will focus on some following parts:

- *Chapter 3: Banana Smoothies*
- *Chapter 4: Blueberry Smoothies*
- *Chapter 5: Green Smoothies*
- *Chapter 6: Mango Smoothies*
- *Chapter 7: Fruits Smoothies*

I want to congratulate you one more time on holding in your hands strategies that can help you *stay healthy, keep you socially and intellectually* engaged in the world around you, and create a living situation that is *comfortable and safe.*

At the bottom line, remember that:

"Happiness lies first of all in health." - George William Curtis

Chapter 1: Top 10 Benefits of Smoothies

✳✳✳

Sixty years ago an American who made it to 65 could expect to live an additional 14 years. Today, it's 19 years. I totally agree with Bob Barker's opinion that age as a number is not nearly as important as health. You can be in poor health and be pretty miserable at 40 or 50. If you're in good health, you can enjoy things into your 80s. So the most important question then: how to grow older healthfully so that we can actually enjoy those extra years? The foremost answer I want to tell you is adopting a new healthy eating habit by consuming smoothies day by day.

Smoothie is one of the quickest and simplest ways for you to start a happy and energetic day. Only with a glass of fresh smoothie can you receive a boost of **vitamins, minerals, antioxidants and a lot of other essential nutrients**. The greatest thing of smoothie is that it's suitable for everyone even the busiest people because it just takes you a matter of seconds. Other things you need are just a Nutribullet blender together with some of your favorite fruits and vegetables.

The health of a smoothie depends on its ingredients. You can adjust fruits and vegetable not only according to your taste but according to the advantage you want to gain. Before telling you about unhealthy smoothie in the next chapter, I'll show you information regarding various benefits you can gain when enjoying smoothie. These benefits listed below will surely surprise you:

- ✓ **Reach your own personal health goals**: Smoothie offers you a pour source of nutrition, as it's free from any preservatives or chemicals, especially when you make it at home by yourself. It's an ideal source to fuel your morning and help you stay alert all day long.
- ✓ **Improved digestion**: Like fresh juice, smoothie extracts every drop of goodness from your raw and natural ingredients and then brings it to your body. However, smoothie's better than juice, whether fruits or vegetables, because when blending fruits and vegetables it still remains **fiber**. Fiber plays such an important part in digestion. Soluble fiber, like that found in cucumbers and blueberries dissolves into a gel-like texture, helping to slow down your digestion. This helps you to feel full longer than juice does.

✓ **Weight loss:** Because of containing fiber that can slow down digestion, smoothie may help with weight control effectively. Let's enjoying smoothies day by day and notice the weight dropping off. You will soon have a fit body as you used to dream.

✓ **Anti-inflammatory:** Inflammation, a normal part of immune system's reaction, occurs in human's body to damaged cells, invading pathogens, irritating chemicals, and other negative factors. However, when inflammation occurs chronically, that is for long periods of time, it can become the root of many diseases. To reduce your overall amount of chronic inflammation, it is important to eliminate, or at least limit, the foods that cause it, and increase foods that inhibit inflammation. You can do this by using your smoothies as vehicles for anti-inflammatory foods such as: berry, kiwi, pineapple, especially turmeric which has the spice giving curry its yellow hue. Compounds in turmeric have been found to reduce joint pain in patients with osteoarthritis and rheumatoid arthritis.

✓ **Antioxidant:** USDA scientists analyzed antioxidant levels in more than 100 different foods. Each food was measured for antioxidant concentration as well as antioxidant capacity per serving size. Cranberries, blueberries, and blackberries ranked highest among the fruits studied. It's so lucky because those fruits are also common ingredients of our smoothies

✓ **Heart health:** Heart disease is the most common cause of death in America; one out of every four deaths in the U.S. is related to it. The efficient way of dropping blood pressure & cholesterol levels to optimum healthy levels as well as way of protecting your heart is avoiding unhealthy food, and eating foods rich in nutrients, fiber, and healthy fats. Luckily, all of those healthy ingredients we can use to make smoothie.

✓ **Beauty:** Think radiant skin, hair, and nails. Supply your body with the vitamins and minerals it requires to grow healthier hair and make your skin glow.

✓ **Deeper sleep:** Improving your health by consuming healthy smoothies almost always results in better sleep at night. A deep sleep not only improves your memory but also restores the body as if we have batteries that require recharging.

✓ **Meal flexibility:** You can consume a smoothie at any meal, not just breakfast. No time for lunch, grab or make a quick smoothie.

✓ **Kids like smoothies:** When combining fruits and vegetables in order to make smoothie, you can make use of all vegetables you usually avoid. The delicious flavor of fruits can hide all flavors of veggies. Your kids will end up consuming smoothies without noticing that you've secretly added a lot of veggies the dislike.

And now, are you ready to gain various benefits of smoothies? Let's take a favorite recipe and make a smoothie for yourself. After that, we will continue to find out the secrets about smoothie.

Chapter 2: Top 10 Tips for Better Smoothies

***

1. *Change up the ingredients*. Using different fruits and vegetables will help you get an even amount of nutrients and health benefits from the varying components. I try my best to use what's locally in season. If you're into green smoothies, be sure to rotate the greens every couple of weeks. This will also keep your smoothies new and exciting and prevent smoothie boredom.

2. *Make use of organic fruits*: Use organic ingredients in your smoothie whenever possible, not only to increase nutrition and avoid pesticides, but also for better taste.

3. *Freeze your fruit*: If you want to make smoothies regularly, it's a great idea to stash some fruit in the freezer. Not only will they retain their nutritional value and flavour, they will instantly chill your smoothie, so no need to add ice. Before your bananas have a chance to turn brown in the fruit bowl, peel and slice them, then freeze on a sheet of baking parchment on a tray until solid. You can then store in sandwich bags and throw into your blender whenever you need them. Even fruits that don't usually freeze well, like strawberries and melon, are ok to freeze if you're using them in a smoothie. Most supermarkets now sell frozen smoothie packs, which are often great value and give you a good mixture of fruit.

4. *Be smart when sweetening*: Remove the pits and soak them overnight or for at least an hour before blending. If using a sweetener, stick to the good ones. Honey, maple syrup, and stevia are excellent choices. In the winter you might find your fruits are not as sweet as you'd like, causing your smoothies to not taste the best ever. Try using fruit juice as the base of your smoothie instead of water. High sugar add-ins: pear juice, bananas, grape juice, apple juice, pomegranate juice and yes a few dabs of agave syrup or maple syrup are good choices too.

5. *Make use of healthy fat*: Avocado is ideal for adding creaminess to smoothies. Its mild flavor disguises its nutritional wallop. After removing its skin and pit, you can add a whole avocado to your smoothie, or save

some for the next day. As an alternative, add ice cream, frozen yogurt, or vanilla yogurt for more creaminess. Work your machine back up to its highest speed, and process for 10-20 seconds.

6. *Gain some grains*: For a heart-healthy way to start the day, add some rolled oats or a few spoonful of cooked oatmeal to your creation. We recommend grinding the oats in a blender beforehand so you'll end up with a powder that won't overpower the texture of your smoothie.

7. *Bump up the goodness*: If you're having a smoothie for breakfast or lunch, make it a more rounded meal by adding some protein. A spoonful of protein powder, peanut or other nut butter, or some tofu will blend well with your smoothie and give you an essential protein boost. Contrary to what you may have seen in Rocky, raw eggs are not a good option as we absorb the protein in eggs much better when they are cooked.

8. *Lose some liquid*: If you're not working from a recipe, begin with less milk or water. It's easier to add more soymilk or water after the fact than it is to round up additional veggies.

9. *Start slow*: No need to go all out from the get-go! Begin at the lowest blender speed, then work your way up to higher ones as needed. You won't put as much wear and tear on the blender's motor or the blades.

10. *Choose a right blender*: Nutribullet blender is highly recommended. With its compact size, simple assembly, hassle-free cleanup, and exceptional nutrient extraction power, the NutriBullet is the ideal tool for health-conscious individuals looking to fuel their exceptionally busy lives. The NutriBullet compact design fits easily on any countertop and plugs into any standard outlet. Its unique Extractor Blade twists directly onto all NutriBullet cups, allowing you to extract and drink from the same vessel, which saves time and reduces additional cleanup.

Chapter 3: Banana Smoothies

***

4th of July Blast Smoothie

Ingredients
- 1 cup fresh blackberries, or more to taste
- 5 large strawberries, hulled and halved
- 1 large banana
- 1/3 cup orange juice
- 2 cups crushed ice
- 1 teaspoon white sugar, or to taste (optional)
- 12 fresh blackberries
- Add all ingredients to list

Directions
1. Place 1 cup blackberries, strawberries, banana, orange juice, and ice into a blender in that order, and blend on high speed until smooth, 30 seconds to 1 minute. Pour into 4 glasses and top each serving with 3 blackberries for garnish.

Nutritional Information
- Calories: 73 kcal 4%
- Fat: 0.5 g < 1%
- Carbs: 17.6g 6%
- Protein: 1.4 g 3%
- Cholesterol: 0 mg 0%
- Sodium: 3 mg < 1%

5 Minute Banana Berry Smoothie

Ingredients
- 4 cups ice
- 1 cup strawberries
- 1/2 banana
- 1 cup orange juice
- 2 tablespoons honey
- Add all ingredients to list

Directions

1. Blend the ice, strawberries, banana, orange juice, and honey in a blender until smooth.

Nutritional Information

- Calories: 85 kcal 4%
- Fat: 0.3 g < 1%
- Carbs: 21.4g 7%
- Protein: 0.9 g 2%
- Cholesterol: 0 mg 0%
- Sodium: 9 mg < 1%

Acai Berry Smoothie

Ingredients

- 2 cups orange juice
- 1 banana, sliced
- 1/2 cup acai berry pulp
- 1 pinch white sugar, or to taste
- Add all ingredients to list

Directions

1. Blend orange juice, banana, acai pulp, and sugar together in a blender until smooth.

Nutritional Information

- Calories: 406 kcal 20%
- Fat: 6.6 g 10%
- Carbs: 83.7g 27%
- Protein: 4.8 g 10%
- Cholesterol: 0 mg 0%
- Sodium: 32 mg 1%

All Around Good Smoothie

"This is a recipe I experimented with to try to get a good amount of vitamins, calcium, protein and fiber in my diet. The great part of this is that I don't get bored with it (even though I drink it every day) because I can change the type of fruit I use whenever I

want."
***Serving:** 10 m | **Total Time:** 10 m*

Ingredients

- 1/2 cup nonfat milk
- 1/2 cup fat-free plain yogurt
- 1/2 frozen banana, peeled and chopped
- 2 tablespoons powdered protein supplement
- 1 1/2 tablespoons flax seed
- 1 teaspoon honey
- 1/2 cup frozen strawberries
- Add all ingredients to list

Directions

1. In a blender, blend the milk, yogurt, banana, protein supplement, flax seed, honey, and strawberries until smooth.

Nutritional Information

- Calories: 345 kcal 17%
- Fat: 5.6 g 9%
- Carbs: 55.9g 18%
- Protein: 26.2 g 52%
- Cholesterol: 5 mg 2%
- Sodium: 271 mg 11%

All Fruit Smoothies

Ingredients

- 1 cup pineapple juice
- 1 large banana, cut into chunks
- 1 cup frozen strawberries
- 1 cup frozen blueberries
- Add all ingredients to list

Directions

1. Pour pineapple juice into a blender and add banana, strawberries, and blueberries. Cover and blend until smooth, about 1 minute. Pour into 2 glasses.

Nutritional Information
- Calories: 205 kcal 10%
- Fat: 1 g 2%
- Carbs: 51.1g 16%
- Protein: 2 g 4%
- Cholesterol: 0 mg 0%
- Sodium: 6 mg < 1%

Almond Berry Smoothie

Ingredients
- 1 cup frozen blueberries
- 1 banana
- 1/2 cup almond milk
- 1 tablespoon almond butter
- water as needed
- Add all ingredients to list

Directions
1. Combine blueberries, banana, almond milk, and almond butter in a blender; blend until smooth, adding water for a thinner smoothie.

Nutritional Information
- Calories: 321 kcal 16%
- Fat: 11.7 g 18%
- Carbs: 55.6g 18%
- Protein: 5.3 g 11%
- Cholesterol: 0 mg 0%
- Sodium: 162 mg 6%

Almond Butter Smoothie

Ingredients
- 1 1/2 cups almond milk
- 2 peeled bananas, frozen
- 4 pitted dates
- 5 tablespoons almond butter
- 1 tablespoon ground cinnamon

- 1 tablespoon flax seeds
- 1/2 teaspoon ground nutmeg
- Add all ingredients to list

Directions
1. Blend almond milk, bananas, dates, almond butter, cinnamon, flax seeds, and nutmeg together in a blender until smooth.

Nutritional Information
- Calories: 484 kcal 24%
- Fat: 27.9 g 43%
- Carbs: 58.4g 19%
- Protein: 9.3 g 19%
- Cholesterol: 0 mg 0%
- Sodium: 303 mg 12%

Amy's Healthy Fruity

"This is the type of smoothie that you can throw together quickly for a meal or snack."
Serving: 10 m | Total Time: 10 m

Ingredients
- 1 cup strawberries, hulled
- 1/3 cup frozen blueberries
- 2 bananas, peeled and cut into chunks
- 1/2 cup orange juice
- 1 1/2 cups plain yogurt
- 1 tablespoon soy milk powder
- Add all ingredients to list

Directions
1. Combine strawberries, blueberries, bananas, orange juice, yogurt, and soy milk powder in a blender. Blend until smooth, then pour into glasses and serve.

Nutritional Information
- Calories: 155 kcal 8%
- Fat: 2.2 g 3%
- Carbs: 29.5g 10%
- Protein: 6.2 g 12%

- Cholesterol: 6 mg 2%
- Sodium: 78 mg 3%

Ann's Berry Green Smoothie

Ingredients
- 2 cups frozen strawberries
- 1 1/2 cups warm water
- 2 cups milk
- 1 1/2 cups fresh spinach, or to taste
- 1 cup frozen blueberries
- 1 frozen chopped banana
- 1 tablespoon honey
- 1/2 lemon, juiced
- Add all ingredients to list

Directions
1. Place strawberries in a bowl; add warm water.
2. Blend milk and spinach together in a blender until smooth. Add blueberries, banana, and honey and blend until smooth. Add strawberries-water mixture and lemon juice and blend until smooth.

Nutritional Information
- Calories: 303 kcal 15%
- Fat: 5.7 g 9%
- Carbs: 57.4g 19%
- Protein: 10.3 g 21%
- Cholesterol: 20 mg 7%
- Sodium: 128 mg 5%

Antioxidant King

Ingredients
- 1/4 fresh pineapple, peeled
- 1 Golden Delicious apple, quartered
- 1 small beet, top and bottom trimmed
- 1/4 cup fresh spinach, or to taste
- 1/4 cup mixed berries, or to taste

- 1/2 banana
- 1/2 avocado, peeled
- 3 ice cubes
- Add all ingredients to list

Directions
1. Process pineapple, apple, beet, and spinach through a juicer.
2. Blend juice, berries, banana, avocado, and ice cubes in a blender until smooth.

Nutritional Information
- Calories: 485 kcal 24%
- Fat: 15.6 g 24%
- Carbs: 93.2g 30%
- Protein: 6.4 g 13%
- Cholesterol: 0 mg 0%
- Sodium: 73 mg 3%

Any Way You Want It Kale Smoothie

Ingredients
- 2 cups chopped kale
- 1/4 cup Greek yogurt
- 3 tablespoons peanuts (optional)
- 1/2 cup milk
- 1/2 frozen banana
- 3 frozen strawberries, or more to taste
- 1 tablespoon maple syrup
- Add all ingredients to list

Directions
1. Blend kale, yogurt, and peanuts together in a blender until smooth. Add milk, banana, strawberries, and maple syrup and blend until desired consistency is reached.

Nutritional Information
- Calories: 469 kcal 23%
- Fat: 22.2 g 34%
- Carbs: 56.8g 18%
- Protein: 18.7 g 37%

- Cholesterol: 21 mg 7%
- Sodium: 145 mg 6%

Apple and Kale Smoothie

Ingredients
- 1 cup Nordica 1% or Fat Free Cottage Cheese
- 1 cup unsweetened applesauce
- 1 cup chopped frozen kale or spinach
- 1 small ripe banana
- 1/2 cup water
- 1/2 cup crushed ice
- 1 tablespoon lemon juice
- 1 teaspoon vanilla extract (optional)
- 1/2 teaspoon ground cinnamon
- Add all ingredients to list

Directions
1. Combine cottage cheese, applesauce, kale, banana, water, ice, lemon juice, vanilla (if using) and cinnamon in a blender. Blend on high speed for 2 minutes or until very smooth. Serve immediately.

Nutritional Information
- Calories: 113 kcal 6%
- Fat: 1 g 2%
- Carbs: 18.4g 6%
- Protein: 8.8 g 18%
- Cholesterol: 5 mg 2%
- Sodium: 153 mg 6%

Apple Banana Smoothie

"Thick and healthy fruit drink with apple, banana and orange juice. The frozen banana takes the place of shaved ice and results in a smooth, creamy texture. Serve with dollop of whipped cream for added effect."
Serving: *5 m* | **Total Time:** *5 m*

Ingredients
- 1 frozen bananas, peeled and chopped
- 1/2 cup orange juice
- 1 Gala apple, peeled, cored and chopped
- 1/4 cup milk
- Add all ingredients to list

Directions
1. In a blender combine frozen banana, orange juice, apple and milk. Blend until smooth. pour into glasses and serve.

Nutritional Information
- Calories: 132 kcal 7%
- Fat: 1 g 2%
- Carbs: 30.9g 10%
- Protein: 2.3 g 5%
- Cholesterol: 2 mg < 1%
- Sodium: 14 mg < 1%

Apple Pie Smoothie

Ingredients
- 2 (6 ounce) containers vanilla yogurt
- 1/2 cup pumpkin pie filling
- 1 banana, broken into chunks
- 2 cups apple juice
- 1 teaspoon ground cinnamon
- 1 dash ground nutmeg
- Add all ingredients to list

Directions
1. Combine the yogurt, pumpkin pie filling, banana, apple juice, cinnamon, and nutmeg in a blender.
2. Blend until smooth, about 1 minute. Pour into glasses and serve.

Nutritional Information
- Calories: 389 kcal 19%
- Fat: 2.9 g 4%
- Carbs: 84.9g 27%

- Protein: 10 g 20%
- Cholesterol: 8 mg 3%
- Sodium: 261 mg 10%

Apple Vanilla Smoothie

Ingredients
- 2 small chilled tart apples, sliced
- 1/3 cup skim milk
- 1/4 cup orange juice
- 1/4 banana, frozen
- 2 tablespoons vanilla whey protein powder
- 1 tablespoon flax seeds
- 1 ice cube
- Add all ingredients to list

Directions
1. Blend apples, milk, orange juice, banana, protein powder, flax seeds, and ice cube in a blender until smooth.

Nutritional Information
- Calories: 422 kcal 21%
- Fat: 6.9 g 11%
- Carbs: 53.5g 17%
- Protein: 41.7 g 83%
- Cholesterol: 13 mg 4%
- Sodium: 242 mg 10%

Apricot Date Smoothie

Ingredients
- 2 peeled bananas, frozen
- 3 apricots - halved, pitted, and frozen
- 5 dates, pitted and frozen
- 1 cup unsweetened almond milk
- Add all ingredients to list

Directions

1. Break bananas into pieces; place into blender. Add apricots and dates; pour in almond milk. Blend until smooth.

Nutritional Information

*   Calories: 362 kcal 18%
*   Fat: 2.2 g 3%
*   Carbs: 90.2g 29%
*   Protein: 4.3 g 9%
*   Cholesterol: 0 mg 0%
*   Sodium: 83 mg 3%

Avocado Banana Nut Smoothie

Ingredients

*   1 cup almond milk
*   1 avocado, peeled and pitted
*   1 large banana, cut into chunks
*   3 tablespoons creamy peanut butter
*   2 cubes ice cubes
*   1 teaspoon vanilla extract (optional)
*   Add all ingredients to list

Directions

1. Blend almond milk, avocado, banana, peanut butter, ice cubes, and vanilla extract in a blender until smooth.

Nutritional Information

*   Calories: 806 kcal 40%
*   Fat: 57.2 g 88%
*   Carbs: 66.8g 22%
*   Protein: 18.8 g 38%
*   Cholesterol: 0 mg 0%
*   Sodium: 401 mg 16%

Avocado Blueberry Banana and Chia Smoothie

Ingredients
* 1 cup vanilla-flavored almond milk
* 1 avocado - peeled, pitted, and halved
* 1 cup fresh blueberries
* 1 banana
* 1 cup ice
* 1 tablespoon chia seeds
* Add all ingredients to list

Directions
1. Combine almond milk, avocado, blueberries, banana, ice, and chia seeds in a blender; blend until smooth.

Nutritional Information
* Calories: 643 kcal 32%
* Fat: 35.3 g 54%
* Carbs: 85.6g 28%
* Protein: 8.6 g 17%
* Cholesterol: 0 mg 0%
* Sodium: 182 mg 7%

Back to the Basics Smoothie

Ingredients
* 1 (11 ounce) can mandarin oranges, frozen
* 1 banana, frozen and chunked
* 1 frozen Gala apple, peeled, cored and chopped
* 1 (12 ounce) package tofu
* 1 cup orange juice
* Add all ingredients to list

Directions
1. In a blender, combine mandarin oranges, banana, apple and tofu. Pour in orange juice. Blend until smooth. Pour into glasses and serve.

Nutritional Information
- Calories: 164 kcal 8%
- Fat: 4.3 g 7%
- Carbs: 26.9g 9%
- Protein: 8.1 g 16%
- Cholesterol: 0 mg 0%
- Sodium: 11 mg < 1%

Backyard Berry Bowl

Ingredients
- 1 cup ice cubes, or as needed
- 1 cup strawberries, divided
- 2 bananas, sliced, divided
- 1/2 cup blackberries
- 1/4 cup apple juice
- 1/2 cup blueberries
- 1/2 cup granola
- 1 teaspoon honey, or to taste
- Add all ingredients to list

Directions
1. Blend ice, 1/2 cup strawberries, 1 banana, blackberries, and apple juice together in a blender until smooth, adding more ice depending on your desired consistency. Pour smoothie into a bowl.
2. Top smoothie with remaining strawberries, remaining banana, blueberries, and granola. Drizzle honey over the top.

Nutritional Information
- Calories: 341 kcal 17%
- Fat: 8.3 g 13%
- Carbs: 64.5g 21%
- Protein: 7.1 g 14%
- Cholesterol: 0 mg 0%
- Sodium: 15 mg < 1%

Banana and Brazil Nut Breakfast Smoothie

Ingredients

- 1/4 cup Brazil nuts
- spring water as needed
- 1 frozen banana, cut into small chunks
- 1/2 cup plain kefir
- 1/4 cup puffed amaranth (optional)
- 1 tablespoon cocoa powder (optional)
- 1 teaspoon vanilla extract
- 1 teaspoon honey
- spring water as desired
- Add all ingredients to list

Directions

1. Pour enough spring water over Brazil nuts in a bowl to cover by several inches; soak in refrigerator 8 hours to overnight.
2. Drain Brazil nuts and put them into a blender; add banana, kefir, amaranth, cocoa powder, vanilla extract, and honey. Blend mixture until smooth, adding spring water as needed to reach desired consistency.

Nutritional Information

- Calories: 669 kcal 33%
- Fat: 33 g 51%
- Carbs: 86.3g 28%
- Protein: 20.2 g 40%
- Cholesterol: 0 mg 0%
- Sodium: 87 mg 3%

Banana and Strawberry Smoothie

"This smoothie will leave you feeling refreshed and give you that little extra boost you need to get you through the day. It also tastes great!"
***Serving:** 5 m | **Total Time:** 5 m*

Ingredients

- 1 banana
- 5 strawberries, hulled
- 1 teaspoon ground cinnamon

- 1 cup cold milk
- 1 drop red food coloring (optional)
- Add all ingredients to list

Directions
1. Combine the banana, strawberries, cinnamon, milk, and food coloring in a blender; blend until smooth; serve immediately.

Nutritional Information
- Calories: 262 kcal 13%
- Fat: 5.5 g 8%
- Carbs: 47.1g 15%
- Protein: 10 g 20%
- Cholesterol: 20 mg 7%
- Sodium: 102 mg 4%

Banana Anna

"A sweet, healthy, easy way to make a banana smoothie. You can substitute soy milk if you like."
*Serving: 5 m | **Total Time:** 5 m*

Ingredients
- 1 banana
- 1 1/2 cups milk
- 1 tablespoon honey
- 1/4 teaspoon ground nutmeg
- Add all ingredients to list

Directions
1. In a blender combine banana, milk, honey and nutmeg. Blend until smooth.

Nutritional Information
- Calories: 356 kcal 18%
- Fat: 7.9 g 12%
- Carbs: 61.8g 20%
- Protein: 13.5 g 27%
- Cholesterol: 29 mg 10%
- Sodium: 152 mg 6%

Banana Avocado and Spinach Smoothie

Ingredients
- 1 banana, sliced
- 1/2 avocado, peeled and sliced
- 1/2 cup fresh spinach
- 1/2 cup 1% milk
- 6 ice cubes
- 2 teaspoons honey
- 1 teaspoon vanilla extract
- Add all ingredients to list

Directions
1. Blend banana, avocado, spinach, milk, ice cubes, honey, and vanilla extract together in a blender until smooth.

Nutritional Information
- Calories: 190 kcal 9%
- Fat: 8.2 g 13%
- Carbs: 27.5g 9%
- Protein: 4 g 8%
- Cholesterol: 2 mg < 1%
- Sodium: 45 mg 2%

Banana Banana Strawberry Smoothie

"Banana extract provides this smoothie with a double dose of fruit flavor!"
***Serving:** 5 m | **Total Time:** 5 m*

Ingredients
- 1 banana, broken into chunks
- 1 teaspoon banana extract
- 3/4 cup milk
- 1 (8 ounce) container strawberry yogurt
- 2 teaspoons white sugar
- Add all ingredients to list

Directions

1. Place banana, banana extract, milk, yogurt, and sugar into a blender. Blend until smooth and serve.

Nutritional Information

- Calories: 468 kcal 23%
- Fat: 6.5 g 10%
- Carbs: 88.9g 29%
- Protein: 17.2 g 34%
- Cholesterol: 29 mg 10%
- Sodium: 224 mg 9%

Banana Basil Smoothie

Ingredients

- 2 bananas
- 1/4 cup heavy whipping cream
- 12 leaves fresh basil, or more to taste
- 1 tablespoon maple syrup
- 4 ice cubes
- Add all ingredients to list

Directions

1. Combine bananas, cream, basil, maple syrup, and ice cubes in a food processor or blender; blend until smooth.

Nutritional Information

- Calories: 234 kcal 12%
- Fat: 11.4 g 18%
- Carbs: 34.6g 11%
- Protein: 2 g 4%
- Cholesterol: 41 mg 14%
- Sodium: 15 mg < 1%

Banana Berry Smoothie II

"A delicious and healthy smoothie that will satisfy a sweet tooth."
Serving: *5 m |* ***Total Time:*** *5 m*

Ingredients

* 1 cup milk
* 1 banana
* 3 large strawberries
* 1 tablespoon vanilla yogurt
* 1 teaspoon honey
* Add all ingredients to list

Directions

1. In a blender, combine milk, banana, strawberries, yogurt and honey. Blend until smooth. Pour into glass and serve.

Nutritional Information

* Calories: 280 kcal 14%
* Fat: 5.5 g 9%
* Carbs: 50.8g 16%
* Protein: 10.5 g 21%
* Cholesterol: 20 mg 7%
* Sodium: 112 mg 4%

Banana Berry Smoothie III

Ingredients

* 1 banana, frozen and chunked
* 1 cup frozen raspberries
* 3/4 cup orange juice
* 1/4 cup vanilla yogurt
* Add all ingredients to list

Directions

1. In a blender, combine banana, raspberries, orange juice and yogurt. Blend until smooth. Pour into glasses and serve.

Nutritional Information
- Calories: 249 kcal 12%
- Fat: 1 g 1%
- Carbs: 60.1g 19%
- Protein: 3.7 g 7%
- Cholesterol: 2 mg < 1%
- Sodium: 23 mg < 1%

Banana Berry Smoothie with Truvia® Natural Sweetener

Ingredients
- 1 cup strawberries
- 1 cup blueberries
- 1 banana
- 1 cup fat-free plain yogurt
- 1 cup orange juice
- 1 cup ice
- 1 tablespoon Truvia® natural sweetener spoonable, plus
- 1/2 teaspoon Truvia® natural sweetener spoonable*
- Add all ingredients to list

Directions
1. Add all ingredients to blender. Blend on high until smooth.
2. Enjoy.

Nutritional Information
- Calories: 121 kcal 6%
- Fat: 0.6 g < 1%
- Carbs: 29.7g 10%
- Protein: 4.8 g 10%
- Cholesterol: 1 mg < 1%
- Sodium: 51 mg 2%

Banana Blackberry Protein Shake

Ingredients
- 2 cups almond milk
- 1 cup vanilla Greek yogurt

- 1 cup ice cubes (optional)
- 3/4 cup fresh blackberries
- 1 banana
- Add all ingredients to list

Directions
1. Combine almond milk, yogurt, ice cubes, blackberries, and banana in a blender; blend until smooth.

Nutritional Information
- Calories: 417 kcal 21%
- Fat: 13.1 g 20%
- Carbs: 60g 19%
- Protein: 17.4 g 35%
- Cholesterol: 19 mg 6%
- Sodium: 379 mg 15%

Banana Blast I

Ingredients
- 1 banana
- 1 pinch ground nutmeg
- 1/2 teaspoon vanilla extract
- 1 cup milk
- 2 cups crushed ice
- Add all ingredients to list

Directions
1. In a blender combine banana, nutmeg, vanilla, milk and crushed ice. Blend until smooth. Pour into glasses and serve.

Nutritional Information
- Calories: 119 kcal 6%
- Fat: 2.8 g 4%
- Carbs: 19.6g 6%
- Protein: 4.7 g 9%
- Cholesterol: 10 mg 3%
- Sodium: 54 mg 2%

Banana Blast II

"This banana smoothie is a very nice drink on a nice summer day."
Serving: *5 m |* **Total Time:** *5 m*

Ingredients
- 2 bananas
- 1 cup milk
- 1/4 cup water
- 2 tablespoons brown sugar
- 8 cubes ice
- Add all ingredients to list

Directions
1. In a blender, combine bananas and milk. Pulse until bananas are chopped. Pour in water and brown sugar. Blend until smooth. Toss in the ice cubes and blend until smooth. Pour into 4 glasses and serve immediately.

Nutritional Information
- Calories: 109 kcal 5%
- Fat: 1.4 g 2%
- Carbs: 23g 7%
- Protein: 2.7 g 5%
- Cholesterol: 5 mg 2%
- Sodium: 29 mg 1%

Banana Blueberry Peanut Butter Smoothie

Ingredients
- 1 cup nonfat milk
- 1 cup fresh blueberries
- 5 ice cubes
- 1 banana
- 1 tablespoon vanilla yogurt, or more to taste
- 1 tablespoon natural peanut butter
- 1 scoop chocolate-flavored whey protein powder
- Add all ingredients to list

Directions

1. Combine milk, blueberries, ice cubes, banana, vanilla yogurt, peanut butter, and chocolate protein powder in a blender; blend until smooth.

Nutritional Information

- Calories: 226 kcal 11%
- Fat: 5.1 g 8%
- Carbs: 34.6g 11%
- Protein: 14.1 g 28%
- Cholesterol: 23 mg 8%
- Sodium: 122 mg 5%

Banana Cherry Smoothie

Ingredients

- 1 banana, cut into chunks
- 1/2 cup Greek yogurt
- 1/2 cup milk
- 1/3 cup frozen pitted cherries
- 1 teaspoon honey, or to taste
- Add all ingredients to list

Directions

1. Blend banana, yogurt, milk, cherries, and honey together in a blender until smooth.

Nutritional Information

- Calories: 198 kcal 10%
- Fat: 6.5 g 10%
- Carbs: 31.1g 10%
- Protein: 6.2 g 12%
- Cholesterol: 16 mg 5%
- Sodium: 59 mg 2%

Banana Coconut Breakfast Smoothie

Ingredients

- 1 1/2 cups vanilla-flavored almond milk

- 1/2 banana, cut into chunks
- 1 scoop vanilla protein powder
- 1 tablespoon coconut oil
- Add all ingredients to list

Directions

1. Blend almond milk, banana, protein powder, and coconut oil together in a blender until smooth.

Nutritional Information

- Calories: 492 kcal 25%
- Fat: 19.5 g 30%
- Carbs: 43g 14%
- Protein: 39.8 g 80%
- Cholesterol: 12 mg 4%
- Sodium: 455 mg 18%

Banana Coconut Smoothie Bowl

Ingredients

- Smoothie:
- 1 banana, divided
- 1/2 cup frozen peach slices
- 2 tablespoons unsweetened applesauce
- 2 tablespoons water
- 2 teaspoons coconut oil
- Toppings:
- 1 tablespoon shredded unsweetened coconut
- 1 tablespoon sliced almonds
- 1 tablespoon raisins
- Add all ingredients to list

Directions

1. Blend 1/2 banana, peaches, applesauce, water, and coconut oil together in a blender until smooth; pour into a serving bowl.
2. Slice remaining half banana and arrange on top of smoothie. Add shredded coconut, almonds, and raisins.

Nutritional Information
- Calories: 317 kcal 16%
- Fat: 16.3 g 25%
- Carbs: 45g 15%
- Protein: 3.3 g 7%
- Cholesterol: 0 mg 0%
- Sodium: 9 mg < 1%

Banana Coconut Smoothie

Ingredients
- 1 banana
- 1 cup milk
- 3 fluid ounces unsweetened coconut cream
- ice cubes
- Add all ingredients to list

Directions
1. Blend the banana, milk, coconut cream, and ice cubes in a blender until smooth.

Nutritional Information
- Calories: 520 kcal 26%
- Fat: 36 g 55%
- Carbs: 44.3g 14%
- Protein: 12.6 g 25%
- Cholesterol: 20 mg 7%
- Sodium: 108 mg 4%

Banana Fruit Smoothie

"This is a great way to cool down. Adjust the honey to your personal taste."
***Serving:** 5 m | **Total Time:** 5 m*

Ingredients
- 1 cup pineapple juice
- 3 bananas, sliced
- 1 tablespoon honey

- 2 cups ice
- Add all ingredients to list

Directions

1. In a blender, combine pineapple juice, bananas, honey and ice. Blend until smooth. Pour into glasses and serve.

Nutritional Information

- Calories: 128 kcal 6%
- Fat: 0.4 g < 1%
- Carbs: 32.6g 11%
- Protein: 1.2 g 2%
- Cholesterol: 0 mg 0%
- Sodium: 6 mg < 1%

Banana Hemp Seed Smoothie

Ingredients

- 2 bananas
- 1 cup frozen peach slices
- 2 tablespoons almond butter
- 1 tablespoon hemp seeds
- 2 cups water
- Add all ingredients to list

Directions

1. Layer bananas, peach slices, almond butter, and hemp seeds in a blender; pour in water. Cover and blend until smooth.

Nutritional Information

- Calories: 250 kcal 13%
- Fat: 12 g 19%
- Carbs: 34.9g 11%
- Protein: 5.4 g 11%
- Cholesterol: 0 mg 0%
- Sodium: 83 mg 3%

Banana Lassi

Ingredients
- 2 over-ripe bananas, broken into chunks
- 1 1/4 cups thick plain yogurt
- 1/3 cup milk, or more to taste
- 2 ice cubes
- 2 tablespoons white sugar
- Add all ingredients to list

Directions
1. Blend bananas, yogurt, milk, ice cubes, and sugar together in a blender until smooth.

Nutritional Information
- Calories: 270 kcal 14%
- Fat: 3.6 g 5%
- Carbs: 52.1g 17%
- Protein: 10.7 g 21%
- Cholesterol: 12 mg 4%
- Sodium: 126 mg 5%

Banana Mint Slush

Ingredients
- 1 cup Silk® Coconutmilk, any flavor except chocolate
- 1 banana
- 6 ice cubes
- 6 mint leaves
- Zest of 1 lime
- Add all ingredients to list

Directions
1. Combine all ingredients in a blender. Blend until smooth.
2. Garnish with mint and lime zest.

Nutritional Information
- Calories: 187 kcal 9%

- Fat: 5.4 g 8%
- Carbs: 34.8g 11%
- Protein: 1.4 g 3%
- Cholesterol: 0 mg 0%
- Sodium: 50 mg 2%

Banana Mocha Protein Shake

Ingredients

- 1 chopped frozen banana
- 1/2 cup chilled brewed coffee
- 1/2 cup unsweetened vanilla-flavored almond milk
- 1/2 cup fresh spinach (optional)
- 1 scoop vanilla protein powder
- 1/2 teaspoon unsweetened cocoa powder
- 1 packet stevia sweetener, or more to taste (optional)
- Add all ingredients to list

Directions

1. Place banana in a blender. Add coffee, almond milk, spinach, protein powder, cocoa powder, and stevia sweetener; blend until smooth.

Nutritional Information

- Calories: 336 kcal 17%
- Fat: 3.2 g 5%
- Carbs: 41.3g 13%
- Protein: 40.1 g 80%
- Cholesterol: 12 mg 4%
- Sodium: 309 mg 12%

Banana Orange and Ginger Smoothie

Ingredients

- 1 orange, peeled
- 1/2 banana
- 3 ice cubes
- 2 teaspoons honey
- 1/2 teaspoon grated fresh ginger root, or to taste

- 1/2 cup plain yogurt
- Add all ingredients to list

Directions

1. Layer orange, banana, ice cubes, honey, and ginger in the blender; top with yogurt. Blend until smooth.

Nutritional Information

- Calories: 176 kcal 9%
- Fat: 2.1 g 3%
- Carbs: 34.6g 11%
- Protein: 7.1 g 14%
- Cholesterol: 7 mg 2%
- Sodium: 89 mg 4%

Banana Orange Smoothie

Ingredients

- 1 banana, peeled
- 1 large orange, peeled and seeded
- 2 cups vanilla-flavored soy milk
- 1 teaspoon ground ginger
- Add all ingredients to list

Directions

1. Place banana, orange, soy milk, and ginger in an electric blender. Process until ingredients are blended and smooth.

Nutritional Information

- Calories: 230 kcal 12%
- Fat: 4.6 g 7%
- Carbs: 40.2g 13%
- Protein: 9.5 g 19%
- Cholesterol: 0 mg 0%
- Sodium: 125 mg 5%

Banana Orange Swirly Goodness

Ingredients
- 2 frozen bananas, peeled and cut into chunks
- 1 orange - peeled, segmented, and seeded
- 1 (8 ounce) container raspberry yogurt
- 1 1/2 tablespoons honey
- 1/2 teaspoon ground nutmeg
- Add all ingredients to list

Directions
1. In a blender, blend the bananas, orange, raspberry yogurt, honey, and nutmeg until smooth.

Nutritional Information
- Calories: 158 kcal 8%
- Fat: 0.9 g 1%
- Carbs: 36.8g 12%
- Protein: 3.1 g 6%
- Cholesterol: 4 mg 1%
- Sodium: 41 mg 2%

Banana Peanut Butter Smoothie

Ingredients
- 1 cup unsweetened almond milk
- 1 frozen banana, sliced
- 1/2 cup ice, or as needed
- 2 tablespoons powdered peanut butter
- 1 tablespoon cocoa powder
- 1 teaspoon cinnamon
- Add all ingredients to list

Directions
1. Blend almond milk, banana, ice, peanut butter, cocoa powder, and cinnamon together in a blender until smooth.

Nutritional Information
- Calories: 232 kcal 12%
- Fat: 4.8 g 7%
- Carbs: 46.3g 15%
- Protein: 7.5 g 15%
- Cholesterol: 0 mg 0%
- Sodium: 236 mg 9%

Banana Pina Colada Smoothie

Ingredients
- 1 large banana
- 1 cup coconut juice blend, or more to taste
- 2 pineapple spears
- 3 cubes ice
- 1 tablespoon agave nectar
- Add all ingredients to list

Directions
1. Blend banana, coconut juice blend, pineapple, ice, and agave nectar together in a blender until smooth.

Nutritional Information
- Calories: 520 kcal 26%
- Fat: 7.1 g 11%
- Carbs: 121.5g 39%
- Protein: 2.1 g 4%
- Cholesterol: 0 mg 0%
- Sodium: 92 mg 4%

Banana Pineapple Green Blend

Ingredients
- 1 cup vanilla soy milk
- 1/2 cup baby spinach leaves
- 1/2 cup water
- 1/2 cup sliced frozen banana
- 1/2 cup chopped frozen pineapple

- Add all ingredients to list

Directions

1. Blend soy milk and spinach together in a blender until spinach is pureed. Add water, banana, and pineapple; blend until smooth.

Nutritional Information

- Calories: 224 kcal 11%
- Fat: 4.1 g 6%
- Carbs: 40.7g 13%
- Protein: 8.2 g 16%
- Cholesterol: 0 mg 0%
- Sodium: 125 mg 5%

Banana Smoothie I

"My father taught me how to make this recipe when I was a little girl. It is very easy to make. This recipe contains raw eggs. We recommend that pregnant women, young children, the elderly and the infirm do not consume raw eggs."
Serving: 5 m | Total Time: 5 m

Ingredients

- 1 banana
- 1 cup milk
- 1 teaspoon vanilla extract
- 1 egg
- 2 tablespoons white sugar
- 1 pinch ground cinnamon
- Add all ingredients to list

Directions

1. In a blender, combine banana, milk, vanilla, egg and sugar. Blend until smooth. Pour into a tall glass and top with a pinch of cinnamon.

Nutritional Information

- Calories: 410 kcal 21%
- Fat: 10.2 g 16%
- Carbs: 65.1g 21%
- Protein: 15.7 g 31%

- Cholesterol: 206 mg 69%
- Sodium: 172 mg 7%

Banana Smoothie II

Ingredients
- 1 banana
- 1 cup cold milk
- 1 egg
- 1 tablespoon wheat germ
- 1 tablespoon honey
- 1 teaspoon vanilla extract
- 1/4 teaspoon ground nutmeg
- Add all ingredients to list

Directions
1. In a blender, combine banana, milk, egg, wheat germ, honey, vanilla and nutmeg. Blend until smooth. Pour into a chilled glass and serve.

Nutritional Information
- Calories: 404 kcal 20%
- Fat: 11.1 g 17%
- Carbs: 60.7g 20%
- Protein: 17.4 g 35%
- Cholesterol: 206 mg 69%
- Sodium: 173 mg 7%

Banana Split Smoothie

Ingredients
- 1/4 cup rolled oats
- 1 tablespoon chia seeds (optional)
- 1 cup pineapple juice
- 1/2 cup chocolate-flavored soy milk
- 8 chunks frozen pineapple
- 6 frozen whole strawberries
- 1 small banana

- Add all ingredients to list

Directions
1. Blend oats and chia seeds in a blender until powdery; add pineapple juice, chocolate soy milk, pineapple chunks, strawberries, and banana and blend until smooth.

Nutritional Information
- Calories: 463 kcal 23%
- Fat: 4.6 g 7%
- Carbs: 101.7g 33%
- Protein: 10.1 g 20%
- Cholesterol: 0 mg 0%
- Sodium: 72 mg 3%

Banana Walnut Smoothie

Ingredients
- 2 bananas
- 1 cup frozen pineapple chunks
- 2 tablespoons cashew butter
- 2 tablespoons chopped walnuts
- 2 cups water, or as needed
- Add all ingredients to list

Directions
1. Combine bananas, pineapple, cashew butter, and walnuts in a blender. Add water and blend until smooth, adding more water for a thinner smoothie.

Nutritional Information
- Calories: 289 kcal 14%
- Fat: 13.2 g 20%
- Carbs: 43.2g 14%
- Protein: 5.7 g 11%
- Cholesterol: 0 mg 0%
- Sodium: 108 mg 4%

Bananerberry Smoothie

Ingredients
- 1 cup fresh strawberries
- 1 banana, sliced
- 1 cup fresh peaches
- 1 cup apples
- 1 1/2 cups vanilla ice cream
- 1 1/2 cups ice cubes
- 1/2 cup milk
- Add all ingredients to list

Directions
1. In a blender combine strawberries, banana, peaches, apples, and ice cream. Blend until smooth. Add ice, pour in milk and blend again until smooth. Serve immediately.

Nutritional Information
- Calories: 354 kcal 18%
- Fat: 12.6 g 19%
- Carbs: 57.8g 19%
- Protein: 6.8 g 14%
- Cholesterol: 48 mg 16%
- Sodium: 114 mg 5%

Basic Fruit Smoothie

"This is a great smoothie consisting of fruit, fruit juice and ice. I like to use whatever fresh fruits I crave that day. Any kind of berry, mangos, papayas, kiwi fruit, et cetera make a great smoothie. Experiment with your favorites!"
Serving: *5 m |* **Total Time:** *5 m*

Ingredients
- 1 quart strawberries, hulled
- 1 banana, broken into chunks
- 2 peaches
- 1 cup orange-peach-mango juice
- 2 cups ice
- Add all ingredients to list

Directions

1. In a blender, combine strawberries, banana and peaches. Blend until fruit is pureed. Blend in the juice. Add ice and blend to desired consistency. Pour into glasses and serve.

Nutritional Information

- Calories: 118 kcal 6%
- Fat: 0.6 g < 1%
- Carbs: 28.5g 9%
- Protein: 1.6 g 3%
- Cholesterol: 0 mg 0%
- Sodium: 16 mg < 1%

Berry Apricot Smoothie

Ingredients

- 1 1/2 cups Original Unsweetened Almond Breeze Almondmilk
- 1/2 banana
- 1 cup mixed frozen berries
- 2 fresh apricots, pitted
- 1 tablespoon chia seeds
- 1 scoop protein powder
- Add all ingredients to list

Directions

1. Place all ingredients into blender and blend on high until smooth.

Nutritional Information

- Calories: 198 kcal 10%
- Fat: 4.5 g 7%
- Carbs: 31.4g 10%
- Protein: 10.8 g 22%
- Cholesterol: 0 mg 0%
- Sodium: 191 mg 8%

Berry Banana and Almond Butter Bliss Smoothie

Ingredients
- 2 cups frozen mixed berries
- 2 frozen bananas
- 2 cups almond milk, or more as needed
- 2 tablespoons almond butter
- 2 teaspoons ground cinnamon
- 1 cup frozen pitted cherries
- Add all ingredients to list

Directions
1. Combine mixed berries, bananas, almond milk, almond butter, and cinnamon in a blender; blend, adding more almond milk for a thinner smoothie, until smooth and creamy. Add cherries and continue blending until smooth.

Nutritional Information
- Calories: 378 kcal 19%
- Fat: 13.7 g 21%
- Carbs: 64.6g 21%
- Protein: 6.8 g 14%
- Cholesterol: 0 mg 0%
- Sodium: 235 mg 9%

Berry Coconut Smoothie

Ingredients
- 1 banana
- 1/2 cup frozen blueberries
- 1 tablespoon almond butter
- 1 tablespoon unsweetened flaked coconut
- 1/2 cup water, or as needed
- Add all ingredients to list

Directions
1. Layer banana, blueberries, almond butter, coconut, and water in a blender; blend until smooth, adding more water for a thinner smoothie.

Nutritional Information
- Calories: 286 kcal 14%
- Fat: 13.9 g 21%
- Carbs: 42.2g 14%
- Protein: 4.6 g 9%
- Cholesterol: 0 mg 0%
- Sodium: 80 mg 3%

Berry Delicious

"After much experimentation I finally got this smoothie recipe right. Frozen berries, strawberry yogurt and a whole banana are pureed in blender for a delicious, drinkable treat."
Serving: 5 m | Total Time: 5 m

Ingredients
- 2 cups frozen mixed berries
- 1 cup strawberry flavored yogurt
- 1 banana, sliced
- 1 cup milk
- 1/2 teaspoon white sugar (optional)
- Add all ingredients to list

Directions
1. In the container of a blender, combine the mixed berries, strawberry yogurt, banana, milk and sugar. Cover, and blend until smooth. Pour into glasses and serve.

Nutritional Information
- Calories: 118 kcal 6%
- Fat: 1.5 g 2%
- Carbs: 24g 8%
- Protein: 4.8 g 10%
- Cholesterol: 6 mg 2%
- Sodium: 65 mg 3%

Berry nana Soy Smoothie

Ingredients
- 1 cup vanilla soymilk
- 1 cup frozen blueberries or frozen berry mix
- 1 banana, sliced
- 1 tablespoon soy protein powder
- 1/2 cup ice cubes
- 1 teaspoon honey (optional)
- Add all ingredients to list

Directions
1. Puree all ingredients in blender on high until smooth. Serve immediately.

Nutritional Information
- Calories: 172 kcal 9%
- Fat: 2.3 g 4%
- Carbs: 33.1g 11%
- Protein: 7.2 g 14%
- Cholesterol: 0 mg 0%
- Sodium: 88 mg 4%

Berry Smoothie Bowl

Ingredients
- Smoothie:
- 1 cup frozen strawberries
- 1 cup frozen pineapple chunks
- 1 cup plain Greek yogurt
- 1/2 cup coconut water
- 2 tablespoons frozen acai berry pulp, or as desired
- Toppings:
- 1 kiwi, peeled and sliced
- 1/2 banana, sliced
- 1/2 cup fresh blueberries
- 1/2 cup fresh raspberries
- 2 tablespoons sliced almonds
- 2 tablespoons granola
- 1 teaspoon chia seeds (optional)

- Add all ingredients to list

Directions

1. Blend strawberries, pineapple, yogurt, coconut water, and acai pulp in a blender until smooth; pour into a bowl. Top smoothie with kiwi, banana, blueberries, raspberries, almonds, granola, and chia seeds.

Nutritional Information

- Calories: 394 kcal 20%
- Fat: 16.8 g 26%
- Carbs: 54.4g 18%
- Protein: 11.2 g 22%
- Cholesterol: 22 mg 8%
- Sodium: 138 mg 6%

Best Smoothie Ever

Ingredients

- 1 (8 ounce) container plain yogurt
- 2 scoops vanilla ice cream
- 8 frozen strawberries
- 1 banana, frozen and chunked
- 1 tablespoon white sugar
- 2 teaspoons vanilla extract
- 1 tablespoon chocolate syrup
- 1/2 cup milk
- Add all ingredients to list

Directions

1. Blend the yogurt, ice cream, strawberries, banana, sugar, vanilla, chocolate syrup, and milk together in a blender until smooth.

Nutritional Information

- Calories: 274 kcal 14%
- Fat: 5.6 g 9%
- Carbs: 46.1g 15%
- Protein: 9.7 g 19%
- Cholesterol: 21 mg 7%
- Sodium: 130 mg 5%

Blueberry Banana and Peanut Butter Smoothie

"This is the perfect smoothie to get your day moving, to give you a boost, or to serve as a kid-friendly snack! "
*Serving: 10 m | **Total Time:** 10 m*

Ingredients
- 1 tablespoon flax seed meal or wheat germ
- 1 banana
- 1/2 cup frozen blueberries
- 1 tablespoon peanut butter
- 1 teaspoon honey
- 1/2 cup plain yogurt
- 1 cup milk
- Add all ingredients to list

Directions
1. Put ground flax seed meal or wheat germ into blender to grind and further breakdown. This will also eliminate any bitterness from the flax seed.
2. Place the banana, blueberries, peanut butter, honey, yogurt, and milk into the blender. Cover, and puree until smooth. Pour into glasses to serve.

Nutritional Information
- Calories: 251 kcal 13%
- Fat: 9.2 g 14%
- Carbs: 34.4g 11%
- Protein: 10.8 g 22%
- Cholesterol: 13 mg 4%
- Sodium: 132 mg 5%

Blueberry Banana Oatmeal Smoothie

Ingredients
- 1 cup soy milk
- 1 frozen banana, sliced
- 1/4 cup frozen blueberries
- 1/4 cup oats
- 1 tablespoon chia seeds

- 1 teaspoon vanilla extract
- 1 teaspoon white sugar, or more to taste
- Add all ingredients to list

Directions
1. Blend soy milk, banana, blueberries, oats, chia seeds, vanilla extract, and white sugar together in a blender until smooth.

Nutritional Information
- Calories: 398 kcal 20%
- Fat: 8.5 g 13%
- Carbs: 68.6g 22%
- Protein: 13.2 g 26%
- Cholesterol: 0 mg 0%
- Sodium: 129 mg 5%

Blueberry Cucumber Smoothie

Ingredients
- 1 frozen banana, cut into chunks
- 1/2 cucumber - peeled, seeded, and cut into chunks
- 3/4 cup buttermilk
- 1/4 cup coconut water
- 2 tablespoons blueberry preserves
- Add all ingredients to list

Directions
1. Blend banana, cucumber, buttermilk, coconut water, and blueberry preserves together in a blender until smooth.

Nutritional Information
- Calories: 252 kcal 13%
- Fat: 2.3 g 4%
- Carbs: 53.5g 17%
- Protein: 8.4 g 17%
- Cholesterol: 7 mg 2%
- Sodium: 264 mg 11%

Blueberry Smoothie Bowl

Ingredients
- Smoothie:
- 1 cup frozen blueberries
- 1/2 banana
- 2 tablespoons water
- 1 tablespoon cashew butter
- 1 teaspoon vanilla extract
- Toppings:
- 1/2 banana, sliced
- 1 tablespoon sliced almonds
- 1 tablespoon unsweetened shredded coconut
- Add all ingredients to list

Directions
1. Blend blueberries, 1/2 banana, water, cashew butter, and vanilla extract together in a blender until smooth; pour into a bowl.
2. Top smoothie with sliced banana, almonds, and coconut.

Nutritional Information
- Calories: 368 kcal 18%
- Fat: 15.6 g 24%
- Carbs: 55.4g 18%
- Protein: 6.8 g 14%
- Cholesterol: 0 mg 0%
- Sodium: 8 mg < 1%

Blueberry Vanilla Graham Protein Smoothie

Ingredients
- 1 cup coconut water, or to taste
- 1 banana, frozen
- 3/4 cup fresh blueberries
- 1/4 cup kale (optional)
- 1/4 cup spinach (optional)
- 2 medjool dates, pitted and chopped
- 1 tablespoon almond butter
- 1 tablespoon hemp seed hearts

- 1 tablespoon flax seeds
- 1 tablespoon oats
- 1 scoop vanilla protein powder (optional)
- 2 tablespoons graham cracker crumbs
- Add all ingredients to list

Directions

1. Combine coconut water, banana, blueberries, kale, spinach, dates, almond butter, hemp seed hearts, flax seeds, oats, and protein powder in a blender. Cover and puree until smooth. Top with graham cracker crumbs.

Nutritional Information

- Calories: 326 kcal 16%
- Fat: 10.4 g 16%
- Carbs: 37.3g 12%
- Protein: 25.1 g 50%
- Cholesterol: 6 mg 2%
- Sodium: 307 mg 12%

BlueCar Smoothie

Ingredients

- 2 cups almond milk
- 1 cup yogurt
- 1 banana
- 1/2 cup blueberries
- 2 pinches ground cardamom
- Add all ingredients to list

Directions

1. Blend almond milk, yogurt, banana, blueberries, and cardamom together in a blender until smooth.

Nutritional Information

- Calories: 435 kcal 22%
- Fat: 9.9 g 15%
- Carbs: 73.1g 24%
- Protein: 17 g 34%
- Cholesterol: 15 mg 5%

- Sodium: 493 mg 20%

Breakfast Banana Green Smoothie

Ingredients
- 2 cups baby spinach leaves, or to taste
- 1 banana
- 1 carrot, peeled and cut into large chunks
- 3/4 cup plain fat-free Greek yogurt, or to taste
- 3/4 cup ice
- 2 tablespoons honey
- Add all ingredients to list

Directions
1. Put spinach, banana, carrot, yogurt, ice, and honey in a blender; blend until smooth.

Nutritional Information
- Calories: 367 kcal 18%
- Fat: 0.8 g 1%
- Carbs: 77.4g 25%
- Protein: 18.6 g 37%
- Cholesterol: 0 mg 0%
- Sodium: 168 mg 7%

Breakfast In A Glass

"A banana is blended with strawberries, milk and yogurt. A delicious way to start the day!"
***Serving:** 5 m | **Total Time:** 5 m*

Ingredients
- 1 banana
- 1/4 cup strawberries
- 1/3 cup nonfat milk
- 1 (8 ounce) container nonfat plain yogurt
- Add all ingredients to list

Directions

1. In a blender, combine banana, strawberries, milk and yogurt. Blend until smooth. Pour into glasses and serve.

Nutritional Information

- Calories: 141 kcal 7%
- Fat: 0.5 g < 1%
- Carbs: 26.3g 8%
- Protein: 9.2 g 18%
- Cholesterol: 3 mg 1%
- Sodium: 112 mg 4%

Breakfast Power Smoothie

Ingredients

- 1 cup So Delicious® Dairy Free Unsweetened Coconut Milk
- 1 1/2 cups frozen strawberries
- 2 bananas, peeled and chopped
- 1 packet vanilla-flavored natural vegan protein powder (such as Vega)
- Add all ingredients to list

Directions

1. Combine all ingredients into a blender, and blend until smooth. Enjoy!

Nutritional Information

- Calories: 608 kcal 30%
- Fat: 7.8 g 12%
- Carbs: 90.1g 29%
- Protein: 54.6 g 109%
- Cholesterol: 17 mg 6%
- Sodium: 305 mg 12%

Breakfast Shake

Ingredients

- 1/4 cup rolled oats
- 1 tablespoon almonds
- 1 cup vanilla-flavored soy milk

- 1 banana
- 1 tablespoon cacao powder
- 1 tablespoon cocoa powder
- Add all ingredients to list

Directions

1. Grind oats and almonds to a flour-like consistency using a coffee grinder. Blend soy milk and banana in a blender. Add ground oats and almonds, cacao powder, and cocoa powder; blend until smooth, 30 seconds to 1 minute.

Nutritional Information

- Calories: 382 kcal 19%
- Fat: 12.9 g 20%
- Carbs: 58.8g 19%
- Protein: 14.1 g 28%
- Cholesterol: 0 mg 0%
- Sodium: 120 mg 5%

Caribbean Health Drink

Ingredients

- 1 cup chopped carrot
- 1 banana
- 1 kiwi, peeled
- 1 apple - peeled, cored, and sliced
- 1 cup chopped pineapple
- 1 cup ice cubes
- Add all ingredients to list

Directions

1. Blend the carrot, banana, kiwi, apple, pineapple, and ice cubes in a blender until smooth.

Nutritional Information

- Calories: 178 kcal 9%
- Fat: 0.8 g 1%
- Carbs: 45.4g 15%
- Protein: 2.3 g 5%
- Cholesterol: 0 mg 0%

- Sodium: 51 mg 2%

Cherry Almond Smoothie

Ingredients
- 1 (8 ounce) container cherry yogurt
- 1 (11 ounce) can mandarin oranges, drained
- 1/2 banana, peeled and sliced
- 1/4 cup half-and-half cream
- 1 teaspoon almond extract
- Add all ingredients to list

Directions
1. In a blender, mix yogurt, oranges, banana, half-and-half and almond extract. Blend until smooth.

Nutritional Information
- Calories: 239 kcal 12%
- Fat: 4.7 g 7%
- Carbs: 43.8g 14%
- Protein: 6.7 g 13%
- Cholesterol: 16 mg 5%
- Sodium: 96 mg 4%

Cherry Banana Smoothie

Ingredients
- 1 cup frozen, pitted cherries
- 1 banana, cut in chunks
- 1/2 lemon, juiced
- 1/2 cup low-fat Greek-style yogurt (such as Fage®)
- 6 ice cubes
- 3 drops almond extract
- Add all ingredients to list

Directions

1. Place the cherries, banana, lemon juice, yogurt, ice cubes, and almond extract into a blender. Cover, and puree until smooth. Pour into glasses to serve.

Nutritional Information
- Calories: 151 kcal 8%
- Fat: 2.1 g 3%
- Carbs: 30.7g 10%
- Protein: 6.7 g 13%
- Cholesterol: 3 mg < 1%
- Sodium: 22 mg < 1%

Cherry Berry Coconut Limeade Smoothie

Ingredients
- 1 1/4 cups cherries, pitted and halved
- 1/2 cup chilled coconut milk
- 1/4 cup strawberries, stemmed and hulled
- 1/2 banana
- 1 lime, juiced
- Add all ingredients to list

Directions

1. Place cherries, coconut milk, strawberries, banana, and lime juice in a blender. Cover and blend until smooth.

Nutritional Information
- Calories: 209 kcal 10%
- Fat: 13.1 g 20%
- Carbs: 24.7g 8%
- Protein: 2.7 g 5%
- Cholesterol: 0 mg 0%
- Sodium: 8 mg < 1%

Cherry Vanilla Smoothie

Ingredients
- 1 cup soy milk

- 1 banana
- 3 ice cubes, or as desired
- 3 tablespoons tart cherry juice
- 1 tablespoon agave nectar
- 1 tablespoon flax seed meal
- 1 teaspoon vanilla extract
- Add all ingredients to list

Directions
1. Blend soy milk, banana, ice cubes, cherry juice, agave nectar, flax seed meal, and vanilla extract together in a blender until smooth.

Nutritional Information
- Calories: 372 kcal 19%
- Fat: 7.8 g 12%
- Carbs: 67g 22%
- Protein: 10.7 g 21%
- Cholesterol: 0 mg 0%
- Sodium: 135 mg 5%

Chia and Almond Butter Punch

Ingredients
- 1 cup almond milk
- 1/2 banana
- 1 tablespoon almond butter
- 1 tablespoon chia seeds
- 1 teaspoon ground cinnamon
- 1 pinch ground nutmeg
- Add all ingredients to list

Directions
1. Place almond milk, banana, almond butter, and chia seeds in a blender. Lightly sprinkle cinnamon and nutmeg on top; blend until smooth, 10 to 15 seconds.

Nutritional Information
- Calories: 265 kcal 13%
- Fat: 15 g 23%
- Carbs: 31g 10%

- Protein: 5.4 g 11%
- Cholesterol: 0 mg 0%
- Sodium: 234 mg 9%

Chia Ginger Smoothie

Ingredients
- 1/4 cucumber, roughly chopped
- 1 frozen banana, chopped
- 1 teaspoon grated fresh ginger
- 1 teaspoon chia seeds
- 1/2 cup orange juice
- water as needed
- Add all ingredients to list

Directions
1. Layer cucumber, banana, ginger, and chia seeds in a blender; add orange juice. Blend mixture until smooth, adding water for a thinner smoothie.

Nutritional Information
- Calories: 185 kcal 9%
- Fat: 1.5 g 2%
- Carbs: 43.8g 14%
- Protein: 3 g 6%
- Cholesterol: 0 mg 0%
- Sodium: 12 mg < 1%

Chocolate Banana Peanut Butter Protein Shake

Ingredients
- 6 cubes ice cubes
- 1 cup milk
- 1 banana
- 1 scoop chocolate-flavored protein powder
- 2 tablespoons peanut butter
- 1 tablespoon honey
- 1 teaspoon unsweetened cocoa powder, or more to taste

- Add all ingredients to list

Directions

1. Blend ice cubes, milk, banana, protein powder, peanut butter, honey, and cocoa powder together in a blender until smooth.

Nutritional Information

- Calories: 561 kcal 28%
- Fat: 22.8 g 35%
- Carbs: 66.6g 21%
- Protein: 30.9 g 62%
- Cholesterol: 60 mg 20%
- Sodium: 341 mg 14%

Chocolate Banana Smoothie

"A quick, cool, tasty treat, perfect for a hot summer day!"
***Serving:** 5 m | **Total Time:** 5 m*

Ingredients

- 1 banana
- 1 tablespoon chocolate syrup
- 1 cup milk
- 1 cup crushed ice
- Add all ingredients to list

Directions

1. In a blender, combine banana, chocolate syrup, milk and crushed ice. Blend until smooth. Pour into glasses and serve.

Nutritional Information

- Calories: 279 kcal 14%
- Fat: 5.4 g 8%
- Carbs: 50.6g 16%
- Protein: 9.7 g 19%
- Cholesterol: 20 mg 7%
- Sodium: 122 mg 5%

Chocolate Cherry Banana Breakfast Smoothie

Ingredients
- 3 small frozen bananas (peel before you freeze)
- 2 cups frozen dark sweet cherries
- 2 cups chocolate soy milk
- Add all ingredients to list

Directions
1. Place all ingredients in a blender. Blend on puree (or the highest setting) until smooth, about 30 seconds. Pour into glasses and serve.

Nutritional Information
- Calories: 166 kcal 8%
- Fat: 1.9 g 3%
- Carbs: 37.2g 12%
- Protein: 3.6 g 7%
- Cholesterol: 0 mg 0%
- Sodium: 66 mg 3%

Chocolate Hemp Protein Shake

Ingredients
- 2 cups water
- 1 banana, cut into chunks
- 1/2 cup raw hemp seeds
- 3 chopped pitted dates, or more to taste
- 1 tablespoon cocoa powder, or more to taste
- Add all ingredients to list

Directions
1. Blend water, banana, hemp seeds, dates, and cocoa powder together in a blender until smooth. Refrigerate until flavors combine, 3 hours to overnight.

Nutritional Information
- Calories: 212 kcal 11%
- Fat: 12.1 g 19%
- Carbs: 19.4g 6%

- Protein: 9.8 g 20%
- Cholesterol: 0 mg 0%
- Sodium: 6 mg < 1%

Chocolate Peanut Butter Banana Smoothies

Ingredients
- 2 (3.25 ounce) cups Snack Pack® Chocolate Pudding
- 2 tablespoons Peter Pan® Creamy Peanut Butter
- 2 large ripe bananas, cut into pieces
- 3/4 cup reduced fat (2%) milk
- 1 cup ice cubes
- Reddi-wip® Chocolate Dairy Whipped Topping
- Add all ingredients to list

Directions
1. Place all ingredients, except Reddi-wip, in blender container; blend until smooth.
2. Divide evenly among 4 glasses; top each with 1 serving Reddi-wip. Serve immediately.

Nutritional Information
- Calories: 222 kcal 11%
- Fat: 7.6 g 12%
- Carbs: 30.2g 10%
- Protein: 4 g 8%
- Cholesterol: 8 mg 3%
- Sodium: 114 mg 5%

Chocolate Strawberry and Banana Smoothie

Ingredients
- 1 cup chocolate soy milk
- 1 cup plain Greek-style yogurt
- 1 cup frozen banana chunks
- 1/2 cup strawberries
- 1 tablespoon ground flax seed
- 1 teaspoon chia seeds

- Add all ingredients to list

Directions

1. Blend soy milk, yogurt, bananas, strawberries, flax seed, and chia seeds in a blender until smooth.

Nutritional Information

- Calories: 559 kcal 28%
- Fat: 26.3 g 40%
- Carbs: 66.7g 22%
- Protein: 19.5 g 39%
- Cholesterol: 45 mg 15%
- Sodium: 265 mg 11%

Chocolate Strawberry Banana Milkshake

"A wonderful milkshake that can easily be adapted for low-sugar diets. My mother got me started on this 20 years ago. I rarely add sugar or sweetener, but I realize that some people enjoy a bit more sweetness. You can substitute orange juice for milk if you like."
Serving: 5 m | Total Time: 5 m

Ingredients

- 1 cup low-fat milk
- 1/2 cup frozen unsweetened strawberries
- 1/2 ripe banana
- 2 tablespoons powdered chocolate drink mix
- 1/2 teaspoon vanilla extract
- 2 teaspoons white sugar
- Add all ingredients to list

Directions

1. In a blender combine milk, frozen strawberries, 1/2 banana, chocolate milk powder, vanilla and sugar. Blend until smooth. If consistency is too runny, you may add more strawberries.

Nutritional Information

- Calories: 139 kcal 7%
- Fat: 2.7 g 4%
- Carbs: 24.6g 8%

- Protein: 4.7 g 9%
- Cholesterol: 10 mg 3%
- Sodium: 61 mg 2%

Chocolate Strawberry Smoothie

"This strawberry, banana chocolate yogurt shake makes a wonderful treat for any occasion."
Serving: 2 m | Total Time: 2 m

Ingredients
- 2 bananas, frozen and chunked
- 1/2 cup frozen strawberries
- 2 tablespoons chocolate syrup
- 1 cup plain yogurt
- Add all ingredients to list

Directions
1. In a blender combine bananas, strawberries, chocolate syrup and yogurt. Blend until smooth.

Nutritional Information
- Calories: 248 kcal 12%
- Fat: 2.5 g 4%
- Carbs: 51.2g 17%
- Protein: 8.3 g 17%
- Cholesterol: 7 mg 2%
- Sodium: 101 mg 4%

Choconananut Smoothie

Ingredients
- 2 cups ice
- 2 cups chocolate soy milk
- 1 large banana
- 2 tablespoons creamy peanut butter, or more to taste
- Add all ingredients to list

Directions

1. Blend ice, soy milk, banana, and peanut butter together in a blender until smooth.

Nutritional Information

- Calories: 315 kcal 16%
- Fat: 9.2 g 14%
- Carbs: 58.2g 19%
- Protein: 10.2 g 20%
- Cholesterol: 0 mg 0%
- Sodium: 82 mg 3%

Chocopeanutbanana Smoothie

"This smoothie tastes like a chocolate, peanut butter, and banana yogurt minus the yogurt. It's fast and easy and good for breakfast. Garnish with a little extra chocolate syrup if you like."
Serving: *5 m |* **Total Time:** *5 m*

Ingredients

- 1 banana, sliced
- 1/2 cup skim milk
- 2 tablespoons peanut butter
- 2 tablespoons chocolate syrup
- Add all ingredients to list

Directions

1. Blend the banana, skim milk, peanut butter, and chocolate syrup in a blender until smooth. Pour into a glass to serve.

Nutritional Information

- Calories: 443 kcal 22%
- Fat: 17.3 g 27%
- Carbs: 63.9g 21%
- Protein: 14.4 g 29%
- Cholesterol: 2 mg < 1%
- Sodium: 229 mg 9%

Cinnapear Smoothie

Ingredients
- 2 pears, quartered and cores removed
- 1 banana, cut in chunks
- 1 cup milk
- 1/2 cup vanilla yogurt
- 1/2 teaspoon ground cinnamon
- 1 pinch ground nutmeg
- Add all ingredients to list

Directions
1. Place the pears, banana, milk, yogurt, cinnamon, and nutmeg into a blender. Cover, and puree until smooth. Pour into glasses to serve.

Nutritional Information
- Calories: 266 kcal 13%
- Fat: 3.8 g 6%
- Carbs: 54g 17%
- Protein: 8.4 g 17%
- Cholesterol: 13 mg 4%
- Sodium: 93 mg 4%

Citrus Healthy Smoothie

Ingredients
- 2 frozen bananas, cut into small chunks
- 2 cups frozen pineapple chunks
- 1 cup fresh orange juice
- 1 cup coconut milk
- 1 lime, juiced
- 2 teaspoons ground turmeric
- 1 (1/2 inch) piece fresh ginger, peeled and chopped
- 1/2 teaspoon ground nutmeg
- ice cubes as desired
- Add all ingredients to list

Directions

1. Blend bananas, pineapple, orange juice, coconut milk, lime juice, turmeric, ginger, nutmeg, and ice cubes together in a blender until smooth.

Nutritional Information

- Calories: 1234 kcal 62%
- Fat: 51.1 g 79%
- Carbs: 206g 66%
- Protein: 11.8 g 24%
- Cholesterol: 0 mg 0%
- Sodium: 49 mg 2%

CJ's Epic Strawberry Banana Smoovie

Ingredients

- 2 cups ice
- 3 frozen bananas, cut into small chunks
- 1 cup skim milk
- 1/4 cup white sugar, or to taste
- 6 fresh strawberries, sliced
- 1 teaspoon pure vanilla extract
- 2 tablespoons whipped dairy topping, or to taste
- Add all ingredients to list

Directions

1. Put ice in a blender; add bananas, milk, sugar, strawberries, and vanilla extract. Blend until smooth. Top with whipped topping; blend again until smooth.

Nutritional Information

- Calories: 166 kcal 8%
- Fat: 0.9 g 1%
- Carbs: 38.4g 12%
- Protein: 3.2 g 6%
- Cholesterol: 1 mg < 1%
- Sodium: 31 mg 1%

Coconut and Banana Smoothie

Ingredients
- 1 cup coconut milk
- 3 scoops vanilla ice cream
- 2 ripe bananas
- 2 teaspoons honey (optional)
- Add all ingredients to list

Directions
1. Blend coconut milk, ice cream, bananas, and honey in a blender or food processor until smooth.

Nutritional Information
- Calories: 414 kcal 21%
- Fat: 28 g 43%
- Carbs: 43.7g 14%
- Protein: 4.7 g 9%
- Cholesterol: 14 mg 5%
- Sodium: 41 mg 2%

Coconut Banango Smoothie

Ingredients
- 1 mango - peeled, seeded, and chopped
- 1 1/2 frozen bananas, sliced
- 1/2 cup coconut milk
- 1/2 cup cold water
- 4 cubes ice, or as needed
- 1 tablespoon white sugar
- 1 teaspoon coconut extract
- 1/2 teaspoon lime zest
- Add all ingredients to list

Directions
1. Blend mango, bananas, coconut milk, water, ice, sugar, coconut extract, and lime zest in a blender until smooth.

Nutritional Information
- Calories: 268 kcal 13%
- Fat: 12.5 g 19%
- Carbs: 40.9g 13%
- Protein: 2.5 g 5%
- Cholesterol: 0 mg 0%
- Sodium: 13 mg < 1%

Coconut Persimmon Smoothie

Ingredients
- 2 ripe Hachiya persimmons, chopped
- 1 cup milk
- 1 banana, cut in chunks (optional)
- 1/2 cup ice
- 1/3 cup shredded coconut
- 1/4 cup honey
- 1/4 teaspoon ground ginger
- 1/4 teaspoon ground cinnamon
- 1/8 teaspoon ground nutmeg
- Add all ingredients to list

Directions
1. Blend persimmons, milk, banana, ice, coconut, honey, ginger, cinnamon, and nutmeg together in a blender until smooth.

Nutritional Information
- Calories: 166 kcal 8%
- Fat: 3.1 g 5%
- Carbs: 34.7g 11%
- Protein: 2.7 g 5%
- Cholesterol: 5 mg 2%
- Sodium: 45 mg 2%

Coconut Raspberry Smoothie

Ingredients
- 2 bananas, broken into chunks

- 1 cup frozen raspberries
- 2 tablespoons pecan halves
- 1 tablespoon coconut oil
- 1 tablespoon flax seed meal
- 1 date, pitted
- 16 fluid ounces water
- Add all ingredients to list

Directions

1. Place bananas, raspberries, pecans, coconut oil, flax meal, and date in a blender; add water. Blend until smooth.

Nutritional Information

- Calories: 373 kcal 19%
- Fat: 14.2 g 22%
- Carbs: 64.8g 21%
- Protein: 3.6 g 7%
- Cholesterol: 0 mg 0%
- Sodium: 11 mg < 1%

Cool Off Smoothie

"Hot and need to cool off? Well, Try my recipe and you'll be cool in no time!"
***Serving:** 5 m | **Total Time:** 5 m*

Ingredients

- 2 cups strawberries, hulled
- 1 cup orange juice
- 1 (8 ounce) container strawberry yogurt
- 2 cups ice
- 1 banana
- Add all ingredients to list

Directions

1. In a blender combine strawberries, orange juice, yogurt, ice and banana. Blend until smooth.

Nutritional Information

- Calories: 214 kcal 11%

- Fat: 0.9 g 1%
- Carbs: 48.3g 16%
- Protein: 6.4 g 13%
- Cholesterol: 2 mg < 1%
- Sodium: 89 mg 4%

Cranberry Orange Power Smoothie

Ingredients
- 1 cup cranberry juice
- 1 large banana
- 1 medium orange, peeled and segmented
- 1/2 cup strawberries, hulled
- 1/4 cup raspberry sherbet
- 1 cup ice cubes
- 1/4 cup whey protein powder
- Add all ingredients to list

Directions
1. Place cranberry juice, banana, orange, strawberries, sherbet, ice, and protein powder in the bowl of a blender. Blend on high speed until smooth, about one minute. Adjust the consistency by adding more sherbet if it's too thin, or more cranberry juice if it's too thick. Pour into two glasses and use a straw!

Nutritional Information
- Calories: 289 kcal 14%
- Fat: 2 g 3%
- Carbs: 54.2g 17%
- Protein: 18.2 g 36%
- Cholesterol: 0 mg 0%
- Sodium: 7 mg < 1%

Cranberry Smoothie

Ingredients
- 1 cup almond milk
- 1 banana
- 1/2 cup frozen mixed berries

- 1/2 cup fresh cranberries
- Add all ingredients to list

Directions

1. Blend almond milk, banana, mixed berries, and cranberries in a blender until smooth; refrigerate until chilled, at least 1 hour.

Nutritional Information

- Calories: 157 kcal 8%
- Fat: 1.7 g 3%
- Carbs: 35.8g 12%
- Protein: 2.2 g 4%
- Cholesterol: 0 mg 0%
- Sodium: 83 mg 3%

Crawford Berry Smoothie

Ingredients

- 1 cup whole strawberries
- 1 cup soy milk
- 1 banana
- 1 tablespoon agave nectar
- 1 tablespoon ground flax seed meal
- 1/4 teaspoon vanilla extract
- Add all ingredients to list

Directions

1. Blend strawberries, soy milk, banana, agave nectar, flax seed, and vanilla extract in a blender until creamy.

Nutritional Information

- Calories: 386 kcal 19%
- Fat: 8.1 g 12%
- Carbs: 72.2g 23%
- Protein: 11.5 g 23%
- Cholesterol: 0 mg 0%
- Sodium: 129 mg 5%

Crazy Fruit Smoothie

Ingredients
- 1 1/2 cups crushed ice
- 1 banana, chopped
- 1 kiwi, peeled and chopped
- 1/2 cup chopped strawberries
- 1/2 cup chopped pineapple
- 1/4 cup cream of coconut
- 1 tablespoon coconut flakes for garnish
- Add all ingredients to list

Directions
1. Blend the ice, banana, kiwi, strawberries, pineapple, and cream of coconut in a blender until smooth; pour into a glass and garnish with the coconut flakes to serve.

Nutritional Information
- Calories: 237 kcal 12%
- Fat: 2.4 g 4%
- Carbs: 57g 18%
- Protein: 3.2 g 6%
- Cholesterol: 0 mg 0%
- Sodium: 23 mg < 1%

Creamy Banana Blast

Ingredients
- 2 ripe bananas
- 1 cup evaporated milk
- 1 cup milk
- 2 tablespoons white sugar
- 2 cups crushed ice
- 1 pinch ground nutmeg
- 4 pinches ground cinnamon, for garnish
- Add all ingredients to list

Directions

1. Blend the bananas, evaporated milk, milk, sugar, ice, and nutmeg in a blender until smooth; pour into glasses and garnish each with a pinch of cinnamon to serve.

Nutritional Information

- Calories: 195 kcal 10%
- Fat: 6.3 g 10%
- Carbs: 29.8g 10%
- Protein: 7 g 14%
- Cholesterol: 23 mg 8%
- Sodium: 94 mg 4%

Creamy Banana Strawberry Split Smoothie

Ingredients

- 1 cup almond milk
- 1 chopped banana, frozen
- 3/4 cup strawberries
- 3 ice cubes
- 1 scoop vanilla protein powder
- 1 teaspoon vanilla extract
- 1 teaspoon honey
- 1 teaspoon ground flax seed
- 1 teaspoon ground chia seeds
- 1/2 teaspoon ground cinnamon
- Add all ingredients to list

Directions

1. Blend almond milk, banana, strawberries, ice cubes, protein powder, vanilla extract, honey, ground flax seeds, ground chia seeds, and cinnamon in a blender until smooth.

Nutritional Information

- Calories: 111 kcal 6%
- Fat: 1.6 g 2%
- Carbs: 14.4g 5%
- Protein: 10.4 g 21%
- Cholesterol: 3 mg 1%
- Sodium: 95 mg 4%

Creamy Pineapple and Banana Smoothie

Ingredients
- 1 cup frozen pineapple chunks, thawed
- 1 cup milk
- 1/2 banana
- 1 teaspoon honey
- 1 teaspoon vanilla extract
- Add all ingredients to list

Directions
1. Combine pineapple chunks, milk, banana, honey, and vanilla extract in a blender; blend until smooth.

Nutritional Information
- Calories: 292 kcal 15%
- Fat: 5.2 g 8%
- Carbs: 53.2g 17%
- Protein: 9.6 g 19%
- Cholesterol: 20 mg 7%
- Sodium: 103 mg 4%

Creamy Pumpkin Pie Smoothie

Ingredients
- 1 frozen banana
- 3/4 cup plain Greek yogurt
- 1/2 cup almond milk
- 1/2 cup ice, or as desired
- 1/4 cup pumpkin puree
- 1/2 teaspoon pumpkin pie spice
- Add all ingredients to list

Directions
1. Blend banana, yogurt, almond milk, ice, pumpkin puree, and pumpkin pie spice together in a blender until smooth.

Nutritional Information
- Calories: 356 kcal 18%
- Fat: 17 g 26%
- Carbs: 42.8g 14%
- Protein: 11.5 g 23%
- Cholesterol: 34 mg 11%
- Sodium: 330 mg 13%

Creamy Strawberry Pineapple Smoothie

Ingredients
- 1/2 cup pineapple juice
- 1/2 cup plain low-fat yogurt
- 1/2 cup halved strawberries
- 1 banana (optional)
- Add all ingredients to list

Directions
1. Blend pineapple juice, yogurt, strawberries, and banana together in a blender until smooth.

Nutritional Information
- Calories: 138 kcal 7%
- Fat: 1.3 g 2%
- Carbs: 29g 9%
- Protein: 4.4 g 9%
- Cholesterol: 4 mg 1%
- Sodium: 45 mg 2%

Creamy Strawberry Smoothie

Ingredients
- 3 cups fresh strawberries, hulled
- 1 medium ripe banana, peeled and halved
- 1/2 cup raw cashews
- 1 tablespoon natural cane sugar (optional)
- 1 1/2 teaspoons vanilla extract
- 1 cup unsweetened coconut milk

- 1 cup ice cubes
- Add all ingredients to list

Directions
1. Place all ingredients in Oster(R) Versa(R) Performance Blender in order listed.
2. Select programmed SMOOTHIE setting.
3. Serve immediately.

Nutritional Information
- Calories: 282 kcal 14%
- Fat: 20.4 g 31%
- Carbs: 24g 8%
- Protein: 4.9 g 10%
- Cholesterol: 0 mg 0%
- Sodium: 120 mg 5%

Currant Affairs Smoothie

Ingredients
- 1 1/2 cups milk
- 1 frozen chopped banana
- 1/2 mango - peeled, seeded, and chopped
- 2/3 cup black currants
- 1/4 cup soft tofu
- Add all ingredients to list

Directions
1. Blend milk, banana, mango, currants, and tofu together in a blender until smooth.

Nutritional Information
- Calories: 215 kcal 11%
- Fat: 5.5 g 9%
- Carbs: 34.7g 11%
- Protein: 9.9 g 20%
- Cholesterol: 15 mg 5%
- Sodium: 79 mg 3%

Dairy Free Chocolate Peanut Banana Smoothie

Ingredients
- 1 cup unsweetened almond milk
- 1 frozen banana, cut into chunks
- 2 tablespoons smooth peanut butter
- 2 teaspoons cocoa powder
- Add all ingredients to list

Directions
1. Blend almond milk, banana, peanut butter, and cocoa powder together in a blender until smooth.

Nutritional Information
- Calories: 369 kcal 18%
- Fat: 20 g 31%
- Carbs: 43.9g 14%
- Protein: 11.3 g 23%
- Cholesterol: 0 mg 0%
- Sodium: 311 mg 12%

Dairy Free Peanut Butter and Banana Smoothie

Ingredients
- 1 cup vanilla-flavored cultured coconut milk
- 1 banana, sliced
- 2 tablespoons peanut butter
- 1 1/2 tablespoons honey
- 1/4 cup ice, or as desired
- Add all ingredients to list

Directions
1. Blend coconut milk, banana, peanut butter, and honey in a blender until smooth, about 1 minute. Add ice and blend again until the ice is crushed, 2 to 3 minutes.

Nutritional Information
- Calories: 572 kcal 29%
- Fat: 24.8 g 38%

- Carbs: 89.3g 29%
- Protein: 9.5 g 19%
- Cholesterol: 0 mg 0%
- Sodium: 163 mg 7%

Dana's Tropical Fruit Smoothie

Ingredients
- 1 (15 ounce) can crushed pineapple with juice
- 1 cup plain yogurt
- 1 banana
- 8 cubes ice
- 1 cup orange juice
- Add all ingredients to list

Directions
1. Combine undrained can of pineapples, yogurt, banana, and ice cubes in a blender. Blend while adding orange juice until fruit is pureed and it is the desired consistency.

Nutritional Information
- Calories: 311 kcal 16%
- Fat: 2.5 g 4%
- Carbs: 68g 22%
- Protein: 8.8 g 18%
- Cholesterol: 7 mg 2%
- Sodium: 92 mg 4%

Delicious Blueberry Smoothie

Ingredients
- 1/4 cup apple juice
- 1 tablespoon instant iced tea powder
- 1/2 cup frozen blueberries
- 1 frozen banana
- 1 tablespoon lemon juice (optional)
- Add all ingredients to list

Directions

1. Place the apple juice, iced tea powder, blueberries, banana, and lemon juice into a blender pitcher. Blend on high until smooth.

Nutritional Information

- Calories: 184 kcal 9%
- Fat: 1 g 1%
- Carbs: 46.2g 15%
- Protein: 2.1 g 4%
- Cholesterol: 0 mg 0%
- Sodium: 5 mg < 1%

Delicious Green Juice

Ingredients

- 1 cup coconut milk
- 1 banana
- 1 mango - peeled, seeded, and chopped
- 3/4 cup fresh spinach, or to taste
- Add all ingredients to list

Directions

1. Blend coconut milk, banana, mango, and spinach together in a blender until smooth.

Nutritional Information

- Calories: 690 kcal 34%
- Fat: 49.2 g 76%
- Carbs: 69.3g 22%
- Protein: 7.6 g 15%
- Cholesterol: 0 mg 0%
- Sodium: 52 mg 2%

Don't Knock it Until You Try it Zucchini Chocolate Banana Nut Milkshake

"I discovered 2 giant zucchini in my garden. I decided to turn this treasure into a challenge and made a whole meal in which each course or dish featured zucchini in

some way. This delicious concoction was what I came up with for dessert. The kids raved about it and asked for seconds."
Serving: *10 m |* **Total Time:** *10 m*

Ingredients

- 1 cup grated zucchini, frozen
- 2 large ripe bananas, peeled and frozen
- 2 tablespoons cocoa powder
- 1/4 cup chopped peanuts
- 1/2 cup sugar
- 1 cup half and half
- Add all ingredients to list

Directions

1. Blend the zucchini, bananas, cocoa powder, peanuts, sugar, and half and half in a food processor until smooth, thick, and creamy.

Nutritional Information

- Calories: 300 kcal 15%
- Fat: 12.1 g 19%
- Carbs: 47.6g 15%
- Protein: 5.6 g 11%
- Cholesterol: 22 mg 7%
- Sodium: 30 mg 1%

Dreamy Cashew Butter Smoothie with Banana Berry Dates and Flax

Ingredients

- 1 ripe banana
- 1/2 cup cold unsweetened almond milk
- 1/3 cup frozen blueberries
- 2 dates, pitted and chopped, or more taste
- 1 1/2 tablespoons flax seeds
- 1 tablespoon cashew butter, or more to taste
- Add all ingredients to list

Directions

1. Blend banana, almond milk, blueberries, dates, flax seeds, and cashew butter together in a blender on high speed until smooth.

Nutritional Information

- Calories: 400 kcal 20%
- Fat: 17.6 g 27%
- Carbs: 59.6g 19%
- Protein: 8.5 g 17%
- Cholesterol: 0 mg 0%
- Sodium: 90 mg 4%

Easy Breezy Coconut and Banana Drink

Ingredients

- 1 banana, broken into chunks
- 3/4 cup milk
- 1/2 cup Greek yogurt
- 1/4 cup oats
- 1/4 cup coconut milk
- 1/4 cup shredded coconut
- 2 tablespoons ground flax seed
- 1 tablespoon white sugar
- Add all ingredients to list

Directions

1. Blend banana, milk, yogurt, oats, coconut milk, shredded coconut, flax seed, and sugar together in a blender until smooth.

Nutritional Information

- Calories: 396 kcal 20%
- Fat: 24.1 g 37%
- Carbs: 38.4g 12%
- Protein: 10.6 g 21%
- Cholesterol: 19 mg 6%
- Sodium: 81 mg 3%

Easy Mango Banana Smoothie

Ingredients
- 2 mangos - peeled, seeded, and sliced
- 2 bananas
- 2 cups vanilla yogurt
- 2 cups milk
- Add all ingredients to list

Directions
1. Blend mangos, banana, vanilla yogurt, and milk in a blender until smooth.

Nutritional Information
- Calories: 133 kcal 7%
- Fat: 2.2 g 3%
- Carbs: 24.4g 8%
- Protein: 5.5 g 11%
- Cholesterol: 8 mg 3%
- Sodium: 66 mg 3%

Easy Power Smoothie

Ingredients
- 1 cup milk
- 2 eggs
- 1 banana
- 1 apple - peeled, cored, and cut into chunks
- 1 teaspoon brown sugar
- 1/2 teaspoon ground cinnamon
- 1/2 teaspoon vanilla extract
- Add all ingredients to list

Directions
1. Put milk, eggs, banana, apple, brown sugar, cinnamon, and vanilla extract into a blender bowl, respectively; blend until smooth, about 30 seconds.

Nutritional Information
- Calories: 468 kcal 23%

- Fat: 15.4 g 24%
- Carbs: 63.9g 21%
- Protein: 22.3 g 45%
- Cholesterol: 392 mg 131%
- Sodium: 244 mg 10%

Easy Pumpkin Pie Smoothie

Ingredients
- 12 ounces vanilla-flavored almond milk
- 8 ounces frozen pumpkin puree
- 1 cup ice cubes
- 1 banana
- 1/2 cup brown sugar
- 1 cinnamon graham cracker, crushed and divided
- 2 teaspoons wheat germ
- 1 teaspoon vanilla extract
- 1 teaspoon pumpkin pie spice
- 1/2 teaspoon ground cinnamon
- Add all ingredients to list

Directions
1. Blend almond milk, pumpkin, ice cubes, banana, brown sugar, 1/2 the crushed cinnamon graham cracker, wheat germ, vanilla, pumpkin pie spice, and cinnamon together in a blender until smooth. Garnish individual servings with remaining graham cracker crumbs.

Nutritional Information
- Calories: 172 kcal 9%
- Fat: 1.7 g 3%
- Carbs: 39g 13%
- Protein: 1.9 g 4%
- Cholesterol: 0 mg 0%
- Sodium: 220 mg 9%

Elvis Smoothie Almond and Banana

Ingredients
- 2 large ripe bananas, peeled and cut into chunks
- 2 cups skim milk
- 1 tablespoon almond butter
- 1 teaspoon vanilla extract
- 1 pinch ground cinnamon
- Add all ingredients to list

Directions
1. Place banana chunks into a sealable plastic bag and freeze until solid, 1 to 2 hours to overnight.
2. Place frozen bananas into a blender with skim milk, almond butter, and vanilla extract; blend until smooth. Pour into a large glass and garnish with a pinch of ground cinnamon to serve.

Nutritional Information
- Calories: 525 kcal 26%
- Fat: 10.8 g 17%
- Carbs: 91.2g 29%
- Protein: 21.9 g 44%
- Cholesterol: 10 mg 3%
- Sodium: 281 mg 11%

Energizing Vegan Mango Banana Chia Smoothie

Ingredients
- 1 mango, chopped, or more to taste
- 1 banana, sliced, or more to taste
- 3/4 cup cold water, or as needed
- 1/2 cup chopped romaine lettuce
- 2 ice cubes
- 1 teaspoon flax seeds (optional)
- 1 tablespoon chia seeds
- Add all ingredients to list

Directions

1. Blend mango, banana, water, lettuce, ice, and flax seeds together in a blender until smooth, about 2 minutes. Add chia seeds to mango mixture and stir. Let sit until smoothie thickens slightly, about 2 minutes.

Nutritional Information

- Calories: 265 kcal 13%
- Fat: 4.9 g 7%
- Carbs: 57.8g 19%
- Protein: 4.3 g 9%
- Cholesterol: 0 mg 0%
- Sodium: 16 mg < 1%

Energy Elixir Smoothie

Ingredients

- 1 cup spring salad greens, or to taste
- 1 cup frozen red grapes
- 1 chopped frozen banana
- 1 cored and chopped frozen pear
- 2 tablespoons walnuts
- water as needed
- Add all ingredients to list

Directions

1. Layer salad greens, red grapes, banana, pear, and walnuts in a high-powered blender; add enough water to cover. Blend mixture until smooth, adding more water to reach desired consistency.

Nutritional Information

- Calories: 421 kcal 21%
- Fat: 11.3 g 17%
- Carbs: 84.7g 27%
- Protein: 6.1 g 12%
- Cholesterol: 0 mg 0%
- Sodium: 27 mg 1%

Fig Smoothie

Ingredients
- 2 frozen bananas, peeled and chopped
- 6 fresh figs, halved
- 3/4 cup milk
- 3/4 cup orange juice
- Add all ingredients to list

Directions
1. Place the bananas, figs, milk, and orange juice into a blender. Cover, and puree until smooth. Pour into glasses to serve.

Nutritional Information
- Calories: 335 kcal 17%
- Fat: 3 g 5%
- Carbs: 77.7g 25%
- Protein: 6.4 g 13%
- Cholesterol: 7 mg 2%
- Sodium: 42 mg 2%

Flax Seed Smoothie

Ingredients
- 1/2 frozen banana, peeled and cut into chunks
- 1 cup frozen strawberries
- 2 tablespoons flax seed meal
- 1 cup low-fat vanilla soy milk
- Add all ingredients to list

Directions
1. Place the banana, strawberries, flax seed meal, and soy milk into a blender. Puree until smooth.

Nutritional Information
- Calories: 273 kcal 14%
- Fat: 8.2 g 13%
- Carbs: 47.1g 15%

- Protein: 7.8 g 16%
- Cholesterol: 0 mg 0%
- Sodium: 121 mg 5%

Fresh Grapefruit Juice Smoothie

Ingredients
- 1 1/3 cups fresh red grapefruit juice
- 8 large strawberries
- 2 medium bananas, sliced
- 1 (8 ounce) container strawberry-banana yogurt
- 2 tablespoons honey
- 1 cup crushed ice
- Add all ingredients to list

Directions
1. Place the grapefruit juice, strawberries, bananas, yogurt, honey, and ice into a blender. Cover, and blend until smooth.

Nutritional Information
- Calories: 361 kcal 18%
- Fat: 1.8 g 3%
- Carbs: 85g 27%
- Protein: 7.2 g 14%
- Cholesterol: 5 mg 2%
- Sodium: 76 mg 3%

Fruit and Yogurt Smoothie

Ingredients
- 1 banana
- 1/2 cup yogurt
- 1 1/2 teaspoons white sugar
- 1/4 cup pineapple juice
- 1 cup strawberries
- 1 teaspoon orange juice
- 1 teaspoon milk

- Add all ingredients to list

Directions
1. Blend the banana, yogurt, sugar, pineapple juice, strawberries, orange juice, and milk in a blender until smooth.

Nutritional Information
- Calories: 147 kcal 7%
- Fat: 1.5 g 2%
- Carbs: 31.3g 10%
- Protein: 4.6 g 9%
- Cholesterol: 4 mg 1%
- Sodium: 46 mg 2%

Fruity 3 Step Acai Bowl Healthy ICE cream!

Ingredients
- 1 banana, broken into chunks
- 1/2 cup almond milk
- 6 fresh blackberries, divided
- 6 hulled strawberries, divided
- 2 ice cubes
- 1 tablespoon coconut yogurt
- 1 1/2 teaspoons acai powder
- 1/2 mango, peeled and chopped, or more to taste
- 1/2 cup granola
- 2 tablespoons shredded coconut, or more to taste
- 2 tablespoons blueberries, or more to taste
- 1 tablespoon almond butter, or to taste
- 1 teaspoon honey, or as desired
- Add all ingredients to list

Directions
1. Blend banana, almond milk, 3 blackberries, 4 strawberries, ice cubes, coconut yogurt, and acai powder in a blender until smooth; pour into a bowl. Top mixture with mango, granola, coconut, 3 blackberries, 4 strawberries, blueberries, almond butter, and honey.

Nutritional Information
- Calories: 780 kcal 39%

- Fat: 36.2 g 56%
- Carbs: 106.8g 34%
- Protein: 15.9 g 32%
- Cholesterol: 0 mg 0%
- Sodium: 178 mg 7%

Gloomy Day Smoothie

"This smoothie is so bright, cheerful, and delicious, it is like a blast of sunshine on even the most rainy, windy days!"
Serving: 10 m | Total Time: 10 m

Ingredients
- 1 mango - peeled, seeded, and cut into chunks
- 1 banana, peeled and chopped
- 1 cup orange juice
- 1 cup vanilla nonfat yogurt
- Add all ingredients to list

Directions
1. Place mango, banana, orange juice, and yogurt in a blender. Blend until smooth. Serve in clear glasses, and drink with a bendy straw!

Nutritional Information
- Calories: 151 kcal 8%
- Fat: 0.5 g < 1%
- Carbs: 34.6g 11%
- Protein: 4.2 g 8%
- Cholesterol: < 1 mg < 1%
- Sodium: 44 mg 2%

Good Morning Green Smoothie

Ingredients
- 2 cups water
- 1 head romaine lettuce, chopped
- 1/2 cucumber, diced
- 1 avocado, peeled and pitted

- 2 stalks celery
- 2 ounces baby spinach leaves
- lemon, juiced
- 2 cups ice
- 1 apple, cored
- 1 banana
- Add all ingredients to list

Directions

1. Blend water, romaine lettuce, cucumber, avocado, celery, spinach, and lemon juice together in a blender on high until smooth, about 30 seconds. Add ice, apple, and banana to blender and blend until smooth, about 30 seconds.

Nutritional Information

- Calories: 151 kcal 8%
- Fat: 7.9 g 12%
- Carbs: 22.7g 7%
- Protein: 3.3 g 7%
- Cholesterol: 0 mg 0%
- Sodium: 46 mg 2%

Good To Go Morning Smoothie

Ingredients

- 2 cups fresh spinach
- 1 cup rolled oats
- 1 cup apple juice
- 1 banana, sliced
- 2 tablespoons peanut butter
- Add all ingredients to list

Directions

1. Blend spinach, oats, apple juice, banana, and peanut butter together in a blender or food processor until smooth.

Nutritional Information

- Calories: 367 kcal 18%
- Fat: 11.3 g 17%
- Carbs: 59.6g 19%

- Protein: 11 g 22%
- Cholesterol: 0 mg 0%
- Sodium: 105 mg 4%

Gordon's Berry Breakfast Drink

Ingredients
- 3/4 cup chilled orange juice
- 1/3 cup chilled pineapple juice
- 2 cups vanilla yogurt
- 1 cup frozen blueberries
- 1/2 cup frozen sliced strawberries
- 1/2 banana, sliced
- Add all ingredients to list

Directions
1. Place the orange juice, pineapple juice, yogurt, blueberries, strawberries, and bananas into a blender. Cover and blend until smooth. The berry drink will be very thick. Serve immediately.

Nutritional Information
- Calories: 120 kcal 6%
- Fat: 1.2 g 2%
- Carbs: 23.7g 8%
- Protein: 4.7 g 9%
- Cholesterol: 4 mg 1%
- Sodium: 55 mg 2%

Granana Smoothie

Ingredients
- 1/2 cup 2% milk
- 1 Granny Smith apple - peeled, cored, and cut into chunks
- 1 banana, cut up
- 2 ice cubes
- Add all ingredients to list

Directions
1. Blend the milk, apple, banana, and ice cubes in a blender until smooth; divide between 2 glasses to serve.

Nutritional Information
- Calories: 113 kcal 6%
- Fat: 1.4 g 2%
- Carbs: 24.9g 8%
- Protein: 2.9 g 6%
- Cholesterol: 5 mg 2%
- Sodium: 27 mg 1%

Green Banana and Peanut Butter Smoothie

Ingredients
- 1/2 cup oats
- 2 tablespoons almonds, or to taste
- 1 cup fresh spinach
- 1 ripe banana
- 2 tablespoons plain yogurt
- 1 tablespoon peanut butter
- 1/8 teaspoon ground cinnamon, or more to taste
- 1 cup rice milk, or as needed
- Add all ingredients to list

Directions
1. Blend oats and almonds in a blender until powdery; add spinach, banana, yogurt, peanut butter, and cinnamon. Blend, gradually adding rice milk, until desired consistency is reached.

Nutritional Information
- Calories: 594 kcal 30%
- Fat: 20 g 31%
- Carbs: 91.4g 29%
- Protein: 18.9 g 38%
- Cholesterol: 2 mg < 1%
- Sodium: 209 mg 8%

Green Breakfast Smoothie

Ingredients
- 2 cups chopped kale
- 1 cup soy milk
- 1 cup fresh spinach
- 1 banana, broken into chunks
- 1/4 cup frozen raspberries
- 1/4 cup frozen pineapple chunks
- Add all ingredients to list

Directions
1. Blend kale, soy milk, spinach, banana, raspberries, and pineapple together in a blender until smooth.

Nutritional Information
- Calories: 377 kcal 19%
- Fat: 5.8 g 9%
- Carbs: 73.3g 24%
- Protein: 15.2 g 30%
- Cholesterol: 0 mg 0%
- Sodium: 208 mg 8%

Green Drink with Aloe Vera Juice

Ingredients
- 1 cup aloe vera juice
- 1/2 cup old-fashioned rolled oats
- 1 cup baby spinach
- 1 cup baby kale
- 1 cup baby chard
- 1 banana
- 1/2 cucumber
- 1/2 cup fresh blueberries
- 2 tablespoons protein powder (optional)
- 1 teaspoon ground cinnamon
- 1 pinch cayenne pepper
- Add all ingredients to list

Directions

1. Mix aloe vera juice and oats together in a bowl; set aside until oats have absorbed the liquid, about 10 minutes.
2. Blend oat mixture, spinach, kale, chard, banana, cucumber, blueberries, protein powder, cinnamon, and cayenne pepper together in a blender until smooth, about 2 minutes.

Nutritional Information

- Calories: 537 kcal 27%
- Fat: 5.2 g 8%
- Carbs: 107.2g 35%
- Protein: 24.3 g 49%
- Cholesterol: 0 mg 0%
- Sodium: 327 mg 13%

Green Monster Smoothie

"Great post-workout snack that will keep you filled for hours! The taste of the banana and the peanut butter cover the taste of the spinach completely. I freeze my bananas and spinach then prepackage everything for the week! Substitutions include rice or nut milks or vanilla yogurt."
Serving: 5 m | Total Time: 5 m

Ingredients

- 1 cup fat-free milk
- 1/2 cup fat-free plain yogurt
- 1 banana, frozen and chunked
- 1 tablespoon natural peanut butter
- 2 cups fresh spinach
- 1 cup ice cubes (optional)
- Add all ingredients to list

Directions

1. Blend milk, yogurt, banana, peanut butter, spinach, and ice cubes until smooth.

Nutritional Information

- Calories: 382 kcal 19%
- Fat: 9.4 g 14%
- Carbs: 55.7g 18%
- Protein: 23.6 g 47%

- Cholesterol: 7 mg 2%
- Sodium: 335 mg 13%

Green Monster Spinach Smoothie

Ingredients
- 1 cup yogurt
- 1 banana, broken into chunks
- 1/2 cup frozen blueberries
- 4 cups fresh spinach
- 1 tablespoon water, or as desired (optional)
- 2 ice cubes, or as desired (optional)
- Add all ingredients to list

Directions
1. Layer yogurt, banana, and blueberries in a blender, respectively. Add as much spinach to blender that will fit; pour in water. Blend on high speed until smooth, adding the remaining spinach if needed. Add ice for a colder and thicker smoothie. Add more water for a thinner smoothie.

Nutritional Information
- Calories: 164 kcal 8%
- Fat: 2.4 g 4%
- Carbs: 29.5g 10%
- Protein: 9.1 g 18%
- Cholesterol: 7 mg 2%
- Sodium: 135 mg 5%

Green Power Mojito Smoothie

Ingredients
- 3 cups ice cubes, or as desired
- 2 cups baby spinach leaves, or to taste
- 1 (7 ounce) can crushed pineapple
- 1/2 cup water, or to taste
- 1 banana, broken into chunks
- 1 orange, peeled and segmented
- 10 fresh mint leaves, or more to taste

- 1 lemon, juiced
- 1 lime, juiced
- Add all ingredients to list

Directions

1. Blend ice, spinach, pineapple, water, banana, orange, mint, lemon juice, and lime juice in a blender until smooth.

Nutritional Information

- Calories: 94 kcal 5%
- Fat: 0.3 g < 1%
- Carbs: 24.2g 8%
- Protein: 1.5 g 3%
- Cholesterol: 0 mg 0%
- Sodium: 19 mg < 1%

Green Slime Smoothie

"This is yummy. With a name like this, your kids will love it."
***Serving:** 5 m | **Total Time:** 5 m*

Ingredients

- 2 cups spinach
- 2 cups frozen strawberries
- 1 banana
- 2 tablespoons honey
- 1/2 cup ice
- Add all ingredients to list

Directions

1. Place the spinach in the freezer until frozen, at least 1 hour.
2. Combine the spinach, strawberries, banana, honey, and ice in a blender. Blend until smooth. Serve immediately.

Nutritional Information

- Calories: 100 kcal 5%
- Fat: 0.3 g < 1%
- Carbs: 26g 8%
- Protein: 1.3 g 3%

- Cholesterol: 0 mg 0%
- Sodium: 16 mg < 1%

Green Smoothie Bowl

Ingredients
- Smoothie:
- 3 cups fresh spinach
- 1 banana
- 1/2 (14 ounce) can coconut milk
- 1/2 cup frozen mango chunks
- 1/2 cup coconut water
- Toppings:
- 1/3 cup fresh raspberries
- 1/4 cup fresh blueberries
- 2 tablespoons granola
- 1 tablespoon coconut flakes
- 1/4 teaspoon sliced almonds
- 1/4 teaspoon chia seeds (optional)
- Add all ingredients to list

Directions
1. Blend spinach, banana, coconut milk, mango, and coconut water in a blender until smooth. Pour smoothie into a bowl and top with raspberries, blueberries, granola, coconut flakes, almonds, and chia seeds.

Nutritional Information
- Calories: 374 kcal 19%
- Fat: 25.6 g 39%
- Carbs: 37g 12%
- Protein: 6.3 g 13%
- Cholesterol: 0 mg 0%
- Sodium: 116 mg 5%

Green Smoothie by Karen

Ingredients
- 3 cups water

- 2 cups packed baby kale
- 2 bananas
- 2 1/4 cups apples, seeded
- 2 3/4 cups strawberries
- 1 1/2 cups frozen blackberries
- Add all ingredients to list

Directions

1. Place water, baby kale, bananas, apples, strawberries, and blackberries, respectively, into a heavy-duty blender. Process on high until completely blended.

Nutritional Information

- Calories: 174 kcal 9%
- Fat: 1.1 g 2%
- Carbs: 43g 14%
- Protein: 3.3 g 7%
- Cholesterol: 0 mg 0%
- Sodium: 23 mg < 1%

Green Smoothie with Maca Powder

Ingredients

- 2 cups chopped frozen pineapple
- 1 cup fresh spinach
- 1 frozen chopped banana
- 1/2 avocado
- 2 tablespoons almond butter
- 1 teaspoon maca powder
- 3 cups water
- Add all ingredients to list

Directions

1. Layer pineapple, banana, spinach, avocado, almond butter, and maca powder in a blender; pour in water. Blend until smooth.

Nutritional Information

- Calories: 330 kcal 17%
- Fat: 17.3 g 27%

- Carbs: 45.3g 15%
- Protein: 5.9 g 12%
- Cholesterol: 0 mg 0%
- Sodium: 100 mg 4%

Green Smoothie

"This doesn't even taste green! Feel free to play with the ingredients. I'm not sure how well other greens go in this smoothie, but the taste of kale is really easy to cover up!"
Serving: 10 m | Total Time: 10 m

Ingredients
- 1 banana, thickly sliced, frozen
- 2 cups chopped kale
- 1 tablespoon flax seed meal (optional)
- 1 tablespoon coconut oil (optional)
- 1/4 cup milk
- 1/3 cup orange juice
- Add all ingredients to list

Directions
1. Place the banana, kale, flax seed meal, and coconut oil into a blender, pour in the milk and orange juice. Cover, and puree until smooth; serve.

Nutritional Information
- Calories: 397 kcal 20%
- Fat: 19.6 g 30%
- Carbs: 53.8g 17%
- Protein: 9.6 g 19%
- Cholesterol: 5 mg 2%
- Sodium: 87 mg 3%

Groovie Smoothie

"Strawberries and bananas are blended with yogurt and milk in this easy and delicious smoothie."
Serving: 5 m | Total Time: 5 m

Ingredients
- 2 small bananas, broken into chunks
- 1 cup frozen unsweetened strawberries
- 1 (8 ounce) container vanilla low-fat yogurt
- 3/4 cup milk
- Add all ingredients to list

Directions
1. In a blender, combine bananas, frozen strawberries, yogurt and milk. Blend until smooth. Pour into glasses and serve.

Nutritional Information
- Calories: 258 kcal 13%
- Fat: 3.6 g 6%
- Carbs: 49.8g 16%
- Protein: 10 g 20%
- Cholesterol: 13 mg 4%
- Sodium: 115 mg 5%

Groovy Green Smoothie

"A great way to get your kids to eat greens! You will be amazed by this yummy fruity smoothie. Experiment with different amounts or types of fruit and make your own."
Serving: 10 m | Total Time: 10 m

Ingredients
- 1 banana, cut in chunks
- 1 cup grapes
- 1 (6 ounce) tub vanilla yogurt
- 1/2 apple, cored and chopped
- 1 1/2 cups fresh spinach leaves
- Add all ingredients to list

Directions
1. Place the banana, grapes, yogurt, apple and spinach into a blender. Cover, and blend until smooth, stopping frequently to push down anything stuck to the sides. Pour into glasses and serve.

Nutritional Information
- Calories: 205 kcal 10%
- Fat: 1.9 g 3%
- Carbs: 45g 15%
- Protein: 6.1 g 12%
- Cholesterol: 4 mg 1%
- Sodium: 76 mg 3%

Hailey's Smoothie

Ingredients
- 3 kiwis, peeled and chopped
- 2 frozen bananas, peeled and chopped
- 1 cup blueberries
- 1 cup plain yogurt
- 1 1/2 cups crushed ice
- 3 tablespoons honey
- 1/4 teaspoon almond extract
- Add all ingredients to list

Directions
1. In a blender, combine the kiwis, frozen bananas, blueberries, yogurt, crushed ice, honey and almond extract. Blend until smooth.

Nutritional Information
- Calories: 194 kcal 10%
- Fat: 1.6 g 2%
- Carbs: 44.2g 14%
- Protein: 4.8 g 10%
- Cholesterol: 4 mg 1%
- Sodium: 47 mg 2%

Hawaii Twist

Ingredients
- 1 small banana, coarsely chopped
- 1 (16 ounce) can pineapple juice
- 3 tablespoons coconut milk

- 1 tablespoon white sugar
- Add all ingredients to list

Directions

1. Slice banana, place in blender, pour in pineapple juice, coconut milk and sugar; blend until smooth. Pour into a glass and serve.

Nutritional Information

- Calories: 476 kcal 24%
- Fat: 10.5 g 16%
- Carbs: 97.4g 31%
- Protein: 3.7 g 7%
- Cholesterol: 0 mg 0%
- Sodium: 16 mg < 1%

Healthier Chocolate Banana Ice Cream

Ingredients

- 1 cup unsweetened vanilla-flavored almond milk, or more to taste
- 1 frozen banana
- 1 tablespoon raw cacao powder
- 1 tablespoon unsweetened coconut flakes
- Add all ingredients to list

Directions

1. Blend almond milk, banana, cacao powder, and coconut flakes together in a blender.

Nutritional Information

- Calories: 160 kcal 8%
- Fat: 6.2 g 10%
- Carbs: 25.5g 8%
- Protein: 2.4 g 5%
- Cholesterol: 0 mg 0%
- Sodium: 82 mg 3%

Healthy Chocolate Smoothie

Ingredients
- 2 very ripe bananas
- 6 ice cubes
- 1 cup milk
- 1 1/2 tablespoons unsweetened cocoa powder
- 1 tablespoon peanut butter
- 1 teaspoon vanilla extract
- Add all ingredients to list

Directions
1. Blend bananas, ice cubes, milk, cocoa powder, peanut butter, and vanilla extract together in a blender on high speed until smooth.

Nutritional Information
- Calories: 229 kcal 11%
- Fat: 7.4 g 11%
- Carbs: 36.7g 12%
- Protein: 8.1 g 16%
- Cholesterol: 10 mg 3%
- Sodium: 91 mg 4%

Healthy Cocoa Banana PB Smoothie

Ingredients
- 1 cup milk
- 1/2 chopped frozen banana, or more to taste
- 2 tablespoons peanut butter
- 2 teaspoons unsweetened cocoa powder
- 1 teaspoon honey
- Add all ingredients to list

Directions
1. Blend milk, banana, peanut butter, cocoa powder, and honey together in a blender until smooth.

Nutritional Information

- Calories: 397 kcal 20%
- Fat: 21.9 g 34%
- Carbs: 39.5g 13%
- Protein: 17.6 g 35%
- Cholesterol: 20 mg 7%
- Sodium: 251 mg 10%

Healthy Fruit and Vegetable Smoothie

Ingredients

- 6 fluid ounces milk
- 1 (6 ounce) container plain yogurt
- 1/2 cup frozen strawberries
- 1/2 frozen banana
- 1/4 cup frozen blueberries
- 1 green ice cube (see footnote)
- 2 tablespoons whey protein powder (optional)
- 1 teaspoon honey, or to taste
- Add all ingredients to list

Directions

1. Combine milk, yogurt, strawberries, banana, blueberries, green ice cube, whey, and honey in a blender, in the order listed. Blend until smooth.

Nutritional Information

- Calories: 372 kcal 19%
- Fat: 6.8 g 10%
- Carbs: 63.2g 20%
- Protein: 18.1 g 36%
- Cholesterol: 26 mg 9%
- Sodium: 358 mg 14%

Healthy Strawberry Smoothie

Ingredients

- 1 cup almond milk
- 1 banana

- 1/2 cup frozen strawberries
- 1/3 cup plain fat-free Greek yogurt
- 3 tablespoons rolled oats
- 1 tablespoon slivered almonds
- Add all ingredients to list

Directions

1. Blend almond milk, banana, strawberries, yogurt, oats, and almonds together in a NutriBullet(R) or blender until smooth.

Nutritional Information

- Calories: 174 kcal 9%
- Fat: 3.8 g 6%
- Carbs: 30.1g 10%
- Protein: 6.4 g 13%
- Cholesterol: 0 mg 0%
- Sodium: 96 mg 4%

Heavenly Blueberry Smoothie

"This blueberry smoothie is to die for! It tastes so good, you forget that it's good for ya!"
Serving: 10 m | Total Time: 10 m

Ingredients

- 1 frozen banana, thawed for 10 to 15 minutes
- 1/2 cup vanilla soy milk
- 1 cup vanilla fat-free yogurt
- 1 1/2 teaspoons flax seed meal
- 1 1/2 teaspoons honey
- 2/3 cup frozen blueberries
- Add all ingredients to list

Directions

1. Cut banana into small pieces and place into the bowl of a blender. Add the soy milk, yogurt, flax seed meal, and honey. Blend on lowest speed until smooth, about 5 seconds. Gradually add the blueberries while continuing to blend on low. Once the blueberries have been incorporated, increase speed, and blend to desired consistency.

Nutritional Information
- Calories: 250 kcal 13%
- Fat: 2.6 g 4%
- Carbs: 50.2g 16%
- Protein: 9.5 g 19%
- Cholesterol: 2 mg < 1%
- Sodium: 117 mg 5%

Holly Goodness Smoothie

Ingredients
- 1 mango - peeled, seeded, and chopped
- 1 small banana
- 1/2 cup frozen raspberries
- 1/2 cup almond milk
- 1/2 cup hemp milk
- 1 teaspoon vanilla extract
- 1 teaspoon chia seeds
- 1 teaspoon hemp seeds
- 1 teaspoon maca powder
- Add all ingredients to list

Directions
1. Blend mango, banana, raspberries, almond milk, hemp milk, vanilla extract, chia seeds, hemp seeds, and maca powder together in a blender until smooth.

Nutritional Information
- Calories: 383 kcal 19%
- Fat: 7.1 g 11%
- Carbs: 76g 25%
- Protein: 7 g 14%
- Cholesterol: 0 mg 0%
- Sodium: 150 mg 6%

Honey Bear Smoothie

Ingredients
- 1 1/2 cups almond milk

- 1/4 cup almond butter
- 2 tablespoons honey
- 1 tablespoon ground cinnamon
- 1 frozen banana, chopped
- Add all ingredients to list

Directions
1. Blend almond milk, almond butter, honey, and cinnamon in a blender until just combined. Add banana and blend until smooth.

Nutritional Information
- Calories: 741 kcal 37%
- Fat: 41.4 g 64%
- Carbs: 93.2g 30%
- Protein: 12.7 g 25%
- Cholesterol: 0 mg 0%
- Sodium: 525 mg 21%

Hot Banana Milkshake

Ingredients
- 2 small ripe bananas, chopped
- 1/4 teaspoon brown sugar
- 1 1/2 cups milk, divided
- 1 tablespoon honey
- 1/8 teaspoon ground cinnamon
- Add all ingredients to list

Directions
1. Mash bananas and brown sugar together in a bowl. Transfer to a small saucepan, place over medium heat, and cook until bananas begin to brown, about 5 minutes, stirring constantly. Gradually mix 1 cup milk into bananas and heat until mixture begins to steam. Stir honey and cinnamon into mixture until honey has dissolved.
2. Pour banana mixture into a blender no more than half full. Cover and hold lid down; pulse a few times before leaving on to blend. Puree until smooth. Blend remaining 1/2 cup milk into mixture until creamy.

Nutritional Information
- Calories: 216 kcal 11%

- Fat: 3.9 g 6%
- Carbs: 41g 13%
- Protein: 7.2 g 14%
- Cholesterol: 15 mg 5%
- Sodium: 77 mg 3%

Jalapeno Green Smoothie

Ingredients
- 2 bananas, broken into chunks
- 2 cups baby spinach
- 1 cup frozen mango chunks
- 1/2 teaspoon chopped jalapeno pepper, or to taste
- 1 cup water, or as desired
- Add all ingredients to list

Directions
1. Layer banana, spinach, mango, and jalapeno pepper in a blender; add water and blend until smooth, adding more water for a thinner smoothie.

Nutritional Information
- Calories: 166 kcal 8%
- Fat: 0.7 g 1%
- Carbs: 42.1g 14%
- Protein: 2.6 g 5%
- Cholesterol: 0 mg 0%
- Sodium: 30 mg 1%

Jumpstart Chocolate Workout Smoothie

Ingredients
- 1 1/4 cups almond milk
- 12 ice cubes
- 1 banana, broken into chunks
- 1/2 cup strong brewed coffee, chilled
- 1/3 cup chocolate-flavored whey protein powder
- 1 tablespoon honey
- 1 tablespoon unsalted natural peanut butter, or more to taste

- Add all ingredients to list

Directions

1. Blend almond milk, ice cubes, banana, coffee, protein powder, honey, and peanut butter in a blender on low speed. Gradually turn speed up to high and blend until smooth, 20 to 30 seconds.

Nutritional Information

- Calories: 285 kcal 14%
- Fat: 7.4 g 11%
- Carbs: 34.4g 11%
- Protein: 22.9 g 46%
- Cholesterol: 60 mg 20%
- Sodium: 234 mg 9%

Kale and Banana Smoothie

"Nutrient-rich kale is hidden in this delicious banana smoothie... perfect for those of us who have a hard time getting our daily dose of veggies!"
Serving: 5 m | Total Time: 5 m

Ingredients

- 1 banana
- 2 cups chopped kale
- 1/2 cup light unsweetened soy milk
- 1 tablespoon flax seeds
- 1 teaspoon maple syrup
- Add all ingredients to list

Directions

1. Place the banana, kale, soy milk, flax seeds, and maple syrup into a blender. Cover, and puree until smooth. Serve over ice.

Nutritional Information

- Calories: 311 kcal 16%
- Fat: 7.3 g 11%
- Carbs: 56.6g 18%
- Protein: 12.2 g 24%
- Cholesterol: 0 mg 0%

- Sodium: 110 mg 4%

Kale and Berries Breakfast Smoothie

Ingredients
- 1 banana, broken into chunks
- 1/2 cup mixed frozen berries
- 1/2 cup shredded kale
- 1/2 cup orange juice
- 1/2 cup water
- 2 tablespoons plain yogurt
- 10 almonds (optional)
- Add all ingredients to list

Directions
1. Place banana, berries, kale, orange juice, water, yogurt, and almonds into a blender. Cover and puree until smooth, 20 to 30 seconds.

Nutritional Information
- Calories: 296 kcal 15%
- Fat: 7.7 g 12%
- Carbs: 56.2g 18%
- Protein: 7.9 g 16%
- Cholesterol: 2 mg < 1%
- Sodium: 42 mg 2%

Kale Avocado Smoothie

Ingredients
- 1/2 avocado
- 1/2 cup frozen mango chunks
- 1 leaf kale
- 1/2 banana
- 2 tablespoons drained canned white beans
- 1/2 cup water, or more as needed
- Add all ingredients to list

Directions

1. Layer avocado, mango, kale, banana, white beans, and water in a blender; blend until smooth, adding more water for a thinner smoothie.

Nutritional Information

- Calories: 314 kcal 16%
- Fat: 15.4 g 24%
- Carbs: 45g 15%
- Protein: 6.1 g 12%
- Cholesterol: 0 mg 0%
- Sodium: 23 mg < 1%

Kale Banana and Peanut Butter Smoothie

Ingredients

- 2 bananas, cut into small chunks
- 1 1/2 cups unsweetened vanilla-flavored almond milk
- 1/2 bunch kale - stems removed and discarded, leaves torn into bite-size pieces
- 4 cubes ice, or more if desired
- 1 tablespoon peanut butter
- Add all ingredients to list

Directions

1. Blend bananas, almond milk, kale, ice, and peanut butter in a blender until smooth.

Nutritional Information

- Calories: 563 kcal 28%
- Fat: 14.6 g 22%
- Carbs: 105.3g 34%
- Protein: 15.7 g 31%
- Cholesterol: 0 mg 0%
- Sodium: 417 mg 17%

Kale Banana Smoothie

Ingredients
- 16 fluid ounces coconut water, chilled
- 1 banana
- 1/2 avocado, peeled and pitted
- 1/2 cup packed kale
- 1/8 lemon, juiced
- 1 pinch cayenne pepper
- Add all ingredients to list

Directions
1. Put coconut water, banana, avocado, kale, lemon juice, and cayenne pepper in blender; blend until smooth, about 30 seconds.

Nutritional Information
- Calories: 371 kcal 19%
- Fat: 16.3 g 25%
- Carbs: 56.2g 18%
- Protein: 7.8 g 16%
- Cholesterol: 0 mg 0%
- Sodium: 510 mg 20%

Kale Orange Banana Smoothie

"Sometimes it tastes like Fruit Loops® cereal, but, of course, this is actually good for you. My 14-month-old loves this for breakfast. Furthermore, he can feed himself (with a sippy cup) while I make breakfast and lunch for the older kids. The texture is similar to pudding. If runnier texture is desired, add ice or milk."
Serving: *10 m | Total Time: 10 m*

Ingredients
- 1 orange, peeled
- 1/2 cup water
- 1 leaf kale, torn into several pieces
- 2 ripe bananas, peeled
- Add all ingredients to list

Directions

1. Blend the orange in a blender until mostly juice.
2. Add the water and kale; blend again on High speed until kale is liquefied.
3. Break the bananas into chunks and add to the blender. Start blending on a lower speed until the banana is incorporated. Increase speed to blend the mixture into a pudding-like texture.

Nutritional Information

- Calories: 220 kcal 11%
- Fat: 0.9 g 1%
- Carbs: 55.9g 18%
- Protein: 3.2 g 6%
- Cholesterol: 0 mg 0%
- Sodium: 15 mg < 1%

Key Lime Pie Smoothie

Ingredients

- 1 1/2 cups ice, or as desired
- 1 (6 ounce) container Key lime-flavored Greek yogurt
- 1 frozen banana, cut into chunks
- 1 tablespoon heavy whipping cream, or more to taste
- 1 splash orange juice
- Add all ingredients to list

Directions

1. Blend ice, yogurt, banana, cream, and orange juice together in a blender until smooth.

Nutritional Information

- Calories: 168 kcal 8%
- Fat: 11 g 17%
- Carbs: 49.2g 16%
- Protein: 14.2 g 28%
- Cholesterol: 37 mg 12%
- Sodium: 108 mg 4%

Kinaja

Ingredients
- 1 cup orange juice
- 2 kiwis, peeled and sliced
- 3 ripe bananas, sliced
- 3 pineapple rings
- 1/2 cup unsweetened pineapple juice
- 2 cups crushed ice
- Add all ingredients to list

Directions
1. In an electric blender, mix together orange juice, kiwi, bananas, pineapple, and pineapple juice until well blended. Pour the mixture into a pitcher.
2. Place the ice in the blender, then pour the fruit mixture over the ice. Process until the ice is blended in with the fruit juices.

Nutritional Information
- Calories: 144 kcal 7%
- Fat: 0.5 g < 1%
- Carbs: 35.8g 12%
- Protein: 1.5 g 3%
- Cholesterol: 0 mg 0%
- Sodium: 7 mg < 1%

Kiwi Banana Apple Smoothie

Ingredients
- 1 apple, roughly chopped
- 1 banana, broken into chunks
- 2 kiwifruit, peeled
- 1 1/4 cups milk
- 1/4 cup ice, or as desired
- 2 teaspoons chia seeds
- 1 teaspoon maca powder
- Add all ingredients to list

Directions
1.   Blend apple, banana, kiwifruit, milk, ice, chia seeds, and maca powder together in a blender until smooth.

Nutritional Information
- Calories: 232 kcal 12%
- Fat: 4.5 g 7%
- Carbs: 44.1g 14%
- Protein: 7.6 g 15%
- Cholesterol: 12 mg 4%
- Sodium: 67 mg 3%

Kiwi Banana Pineapple Orange Smoothie

Ingredients
- 1 kiwifruit, peeled and sliced
- 1 banana
- 1/2 cup orange juice
- 1/2 cup diced pineapple
- 1/4 cup coconut water
- 1/4 cup low-fat vanilla yogurt
- 1 teaspoon agave nectar (optional)
- Add all ingredients to list

Directions
1.   Blend kiwi, banana, orange juice, pineapple, coconut water, yogurt, and agave nectar in a blender until smooth.

Nutritional Information
- Calories: 165 kcal 8%
- Fat: 1 g 2%
- Carbs: 38.8g 13%
- Protein: 3.4 g 7%
- Cholesterol: 2 mg < 1%
- Sodium: 54 mg 2%

Kiwi Strawberry Smoothie

"Fruity goodness for smoothie lovers!"
Serving: *5 m* | **Total Time:** *5 m*

Ingredients
- 1 banana
- 6 strawberries
- 1 kiwi
- 1/2 cup vanilla frozen yogurt
- 3/4 cup pineapple and orange juice blend
- Add all ingredients to list

Directions
1. Place the banana, strawberries, kiwi, vanilla frozen yogurt, and pineapple and orange juice blend in a blender. Blend until smooth.

Nutritional Information
- Calories: 204 kcal 10%
- Fat: 0.5 g < 1%
- Carbs: 48.1g 16%
- Protein: 4.3 g 9%
- Cholesterol: 2 mg < 1%
- Sodium: 34 mg 1%

Kiwinanaberry Cream Smoothie

Ingredients
- 5 kiwis
- 1 banana
- 2 tangelos
- 1 cup mixed fresh berries
- 1 1/2 cups plain yogurt
- 1 1/4 cups soy milk
- 1 tablespoon white sugar
- 1 sprig fresh mint leaves
- Add all ingredients to list

Directions
1. In a blender or food processor, blend the kiwis, banana, tangelos, berries, yogurt, and soy milk. Gradually blend in the sugar to taste. Serve in tall glasses with fresh mint.

Nutritional Information
- Calories: 238 kcal 12%
- Fat: 3.6 g 6%
- Carbs: 45.6g 15%
- Protein: 9.4 g 19%
- Cholesterol: 6 mg 2%
- Sodium: 108 mg 4%

Lean and Green

Ingredients
- 1 cup fresh spinach
- 1 banana
- 1/2 green apple
- 4 hulled strawberries
- 4 (1 inch) pieces frozen mango
- 1/3 cup whole milk
- 1 scoop vanilla protein powder (optional)
- 1 teaspoon honey
- Add all ingredients to list

Directions
1. Blend spinach, banana, apple, strawberries, mango, milk, protein powder, and honey together in a blender until smooth.

Nutritional Information
- Calories: 456 kcal 23%
- Fat: 4.9 g 8%
- Carbs: 66.9g 22%
- Protein: 43.3 g 87%
- Cholesterol: 21 mg 7%
- Sodium: 273 mg 11%

Lemon Spinach Mint Smoothie

Ingredients
- 1 cup fresh spinach, or more to taste
- 1/2 banana
- 1/2 avocado
- 1 kiwi, peeled and ends removed
- 1 lemon, juiced
- 10 mint leaves
- 6 raw almonds
- 1 tablespoon maple syrup
- 1 teaspoon flax seeds
- 1 cup cold water, or as needed to cover
- 3 ice cubes
- Add all ingredients to list

Directions
1. Combine spinach, banana, avocado, kiwi, lemon juice, mint, almonds, maple syrup, and flax seeds in a blender. Add enough water to almost cover ingredients; blend until smooth. Add ice and blend thoroughly.

Nutritional Information
- Calories: 243 kcal 12%
- Fat: 8.2 g 13%
- Carbs: 42.6g 14%
- Protein: 4.9 g 10%
- Cholesterol: 0 mg 0%
- Sodium: 40 mg 2%

Lexi's Protein Packed Smoothie

Ingredients
- 1/2 cup nonfat plain yogurt
- 1/2 cup strawberries
- 1/4 (16 ounce) package silken tofu
- 1 banana, cut into chunks
- 1/4 cup milk, or to taste
- 1 tablespoon white sugar, or to taste
- Add all ingredients to list

Directions

1. Blend yogurt, strawberries, tofu, banana, milk, and sugar together in a blender until desired consistency is reached.

Nutritional Information

- Calories: 170 kcal 8%
- Fat: 2.6 g 4%
- Carbs: 30.5g 10%
- Protein: 8.1 g 16%
- Cholesterol: 4 mg 1%
- Sodium: 63 mg 3%

Mal's Killer Vegan PB and J Smoothie

Ingredients

- 3/4 cup frozen marionberries
- 1/2 cup hemp milk, or more to taste
- 1/4 cup chopped kale, or to taste
- 1/2 frozen banana, sliced (optional)
- 2 cubes ice, or as needed
- 1 tablespoon cashew butter, or more to taste
- 1 tablespoon chia seeds (optional)
- 1 teaspoon honey, or more to taste
- 1 splash orange blossom water (optional)
- Add all ingredients to list

Directions

1. Blend marionberries, hemp milk, kale, banana, ice, cashew butter, chia seeds, honey, and orange blossom water together in a blender until smooth.

Nutritional Information

- Calories: 357 kcal 18%
- Fat: 13.5 g 21%
- Carbs: 56.8g 18%
- Protein: 8 g 16%
- Cholesterol: 0 mg 0%
- Sodium: 81 mg 3%

Mango Banana Smoothie

"I love mangoes and fresh fruit. This is awesome to make and pack to have with you around town in a bottle, or just have for breakfast anytime."
Serving:** 5 m |* ***Total Time: *5 m*

Ingredients
- 1 banana
- 1/2 cup frozen mango pieces
- 1/3 cup plain yogurt
- 1/2 cup orange-mango juice blend
- Add all ingredients to list

Directions
1. Combine the banana, mango, yogurt, and juice in a blender; blend until nearly smooth.

Nutritional Information
- Calories: 135 kcal 7%
- Fat: 0.9 g 1%
- Carbs: 30.4g 10%
- Protein: 3.2 g 6%
- Cholesterol: 2 mg < 1%
- Sodium: 39 mg 2%

Mango Chia Smoothie

Ingredients
- 1 1/2 cups almond milk
- 1 1/2 cups fresh spinach (optional)
- 1 mango, peeled and cubed
- 1 banana
- 1/2 cup ice cubes
- 2 tablespoons chia seeds
- 1 teaspoon honey
- 1/2 teaspoon ground turmeric
- Add all ingredients to list

Directions

1. Blend almond milk, spinach, mango, banana, ice cubes, chia seeds, honey, and turmeric in a blender until smooth, about 30 seconds.

Nutritional Information

- Calories: 409 kcal 20%
- Fat: 9.7 g 15%
- Carbs: 80.3g 26%
- Protein: 7.4 g 15%
- Cholesterol: 0 mg 0%
- Sodium: 287 mg 11%

Mango Oatmeal Breakfast Smoothie

Ingredients

- 1/2 cup orange juice
- 1/2 cup frozen mango chunks
- 1/2 banana, cut into chunks
- 1/3 cup plain yogurt
- 1/4 cup oats
- Add all ingredients to list

Directions

1. Blend orange juice, mango, banana, yogurt, and oats together in a blender until smooth.

Nutritional Information

- Calories: 290 kcal 15%
- Fat: 3.3 g 5%
- Carbs: 59.9g 19%
- Protein: 8.9 g 18%
- Cholesterol: 5 mg 2%
- Sodium: 62 mg 2%

Mango Peach Banana Smoothie

Ingredients

- 1 (16 ounce) can mango nectar

- 1 cup peach yogurt
- 1 cup vanilla frozen yogurt
- 1 1/2 cups frozen peach slices
- 1 frozen banana, cut into chunks
- Add all ingredients to list

Directions
1. Combine mango nectar, peach yogurt, and frozen yogurt in pitcher of a blender; add peach slices and banana chunks. Blend until smooth, 30 seconds to 1 minute.

Nutritional Information
- Calories: 322 kcal 16%
- Fat: 1 g 2%
- Carbs: 74.8g 24%
- Protein: 6.9 g 14%
- Cholesterol: 6 mg 2%
- Sodium: 72 mg 3%

Mango Pineapple Green Smoothie

Ingredients
- 2/3 cup frozen pineapple chunks
- 1 cup frozen mango chunks
- 1 ripe banana, sliced
- 2/3 cup fresh spinach
- 1/3 cup orange juice
- 1 cup ice
- Add all ingredients to list

Directions
1. Place pineapple, mango, banana, spinach, orange juice, and ice, respectively, in a blender and blend until smooth.

Nutritional Information
- Calories: 197 kcal 10%
- Fat: 0.6 g < 1%
- Carbs: 50.3g 16%
- Protein: 2 g 4%

- Cholesterol: 0 mg 0%
- Sodium: 16 mg < 1%

Mango Pineapple Smoothie

Ingredients
- 1 cup vanilla yogurt
- 1 cup unsweetened pineapple juice
- 1/2 banana, sliced
- 1 mango - peeled, seeded, and chopped
- 1/2 cup nonfat milk
- 2 tablespoons cream of coconut
- Add all ingredients to list

Directions
1. In a blender, blend the vanilla yogurt, pineapple juice, banana, mango, milk, and cream of coconut until smooth.

Nutritional Information
- Calories: 178 kcal 9%
- Fat: 2.7 g 4%
- Carbs: 35.7g 12%
- Protein: 4.7 g 9%
- Cholesterol: 4 mg 1%
- Sodium: 61 mg 2%

Marie's Healthy Breakfast Smoothie

Ingredients
- 1/2 cup spinach, or more to taste
- 1 frozen banana, cut into chunks
- 1/2 small avocado, peeled and pitted
- 1/4 cup almond milk
- 1/2 teaspoon vanilla extract
- 1/4 teaspoon ground cinnamon
- Add all ingredients to list

Directions

1. Blend spinach, banana, avocado, almond milk, vanilla extract, and cinnamon together in a blender until smooth.

Nutritional Information

*   Calories: 268 kcal 13%
*   Fat: 13.6 g 21%
*   Carbs: 37.6g 12%
*   Protein: 3.7 g 7%
*   Cholesterol: 0 mg 0%
*   Sodium: 59 mg 2%

Marlene's Yogurt Berry Smoothie

Ingredients

*   1 cup soy milk
*   2 tablespoons flax seed meal
*   1 cup Greek yogurt (such as Chobani®)
*   1 cup fresh strawberries
*   1/2 banana
*   3 ounces baby carrots, cut into chunks
*   1 tablespoon flaked coconut
*   1 cup frozen blueberries
*   Add all ingredients to list

Directions

1. Pour soy milk and flax seeds into a blender. Allow flax seeds to soften, 1 to 3 minutes. Turn blender on and add yogurt, strawberries, banana, carrots, and coconut, blending well after each addition. Add blueberries and blend until smooth.

Nutritional Information

*   Calories: 359 kcal 18%
*   Fat: 17.6 g 27%
*   Carbs: 41g 13%
*   Protein: 13.1 g 26%
*   Cholesterol: 22 mg 8%
*   Sodium: 165 mg 7%

Matcha Berry Swirl Smoothie

Ingredients
- 2 cups fresh spinach
- 2 cups orange juice, divided
- 1 cup frozen peaches
- 1 cup frozen pineapple chunks
- 2 frozen bananas, halved, divided
- 2 teaspoons green tea powder (matcha)
- 1 cup frozen raspberries
- 1 cup frozen strawberries
- Add all ingredients to list

Directions
1. Combine spinach, 1 cup orange juice, peaches, pineapple, 1 halved banana, and green tea powder in a blender; blend until combined. Pour smoothie into a glass.
2. Rinse out the blender.
3. Combine 1 cup orange juice, raspberries, strawberries, and 1 halved banana in the blender; blend until combined. Pour berry smoothie into a separate glass.
4. Combine smoothies by pouring them at the same time from opposite sides of the serving glass.

Nutritional Information
- Calories: 262 kcal 13%
- Fat: 0.7 g 1%
- Carbs: 65.6g 21%
- Protein: 3.3 g 7%
- Cholesterol: 0 mg 0%
- Sodium: 17 mg < 1%

Matcha Coconut Smoothie

Ingredients
- 1 banana
- 1 cup frozen mango chunks
- 2 leaves kale, torn into several pieces
- 3 tablespoons white beans, drained
- 2 tablespoons unsweetened shredded coconut
- 1/2 teaspoon matcha green tea powder

- 1 cup water
- Add all ingredients to list

Directions
1.   Combine banana, mango, kale, white beans, coconut, and matcha powder in a blender; add water. Blend mixture until very smooth.

Nutritional Information
- Calories: 367 kcal 18%
- Fat: 8.8 g 14%
- Carbs: 72.4g 23%
- Protein: 8 g 16%
- Cholesterol: 0 mg 0%
- Sodium: 36 mg 1%

Matcha Smoothie

Ingredients
- 1 cup ice cubes, or as desired
- 1 cup orange juice
- 1 ripe banana
- 1/2 teaspoon matcha green tea powder, or more to taste
- Add all ingredients to list

Directions
1.   Blend ice cubes, orange juice, banana, and matcha powder together in a blender until smooth.

Nutritional Information
- Calories: 218 kcal 11%
- Fat: 0.9 g 1%
- Carbs: 53g 17%
- Protein: 3.2 g 6%
- Cholesterol: 0 mg 0%
- Sodium: 11 mg < 1%

Max's Fresh Fruit Smoothie

Ingredients
- 3 fresh apricots, pitted and diced
- 1 banana, diced
- 1 cup milk
- 4 teaspoons white sugar
- 13 cubes ice
- Add all ingredients to list

Directions
1. Blend the apricots, banana, milk, sugar, and ice in a blender until smooth, thick, and frosty.

Nutritional Information
- Calories: 114 kcal 6%
- Fat: 1.9 g 3%
- Carbs: 22.2g 7%
- Protein: 3.6 g 7%
- Cholesterol: 7 mg 2%
- Sodium: 37 mg 1%

Mega Mango Smoothie

Ingredients
- 1 1/2 cups frozen mango chunks
- 1 cup Nordica 1% Cottage Cheese
- 1 cup ice cubes
- 1/2 cup orange juice
- 1/2 cup cold water
- 1 small banana, cut into chunks
- 2 tablespoons honey
- 1 tablespoon flax oil
- 1 teaspoon vanilla extract
- Add all ingredients to list

Directions
1. Place the mango, cottage cheese, ice cubes, orange juice, water, banana, honey, flax oil and vanilla in a blender. Blend for 2 minutes or until very smooth;

serve immediately.

Nutritional Information
- Calories: 383 kcal 19%
- Fat: 8.9 g 14%
- Carbs: 63.6g 21%
- Protein: 16.7 g 33%
- Cholesterol: 10 mg 3%
- Sodium: 300 mg 12%

Melon Blackberry Smoothie

Ingredients
- 1 banana, chopped
- 1/2 honeydew melon, cubed
- 1/2 cup frozen blackberries
- 3 tablespoons wheat germ
- 3/4 cup almond milk
- 6 ice cubes
- Add all ingredients to list

Directions
1. Place the banana, honeydew melon, blackberries, wheat germ, and almond milk into a blender. Cover, and puree until smooth.
2. Divide ice cubes into two tall glasses, and pour the smoothie over the ice.

Nutritional Information
- Calories: 254 kcal 13%
- Fat: 2.8 g 4%
- Carbs: 57.2g 18%
- Protein: 5.7 g 11%
- Cholesterol: 0 mg 0%
- Sodium: 122 mg 5%

Milk Banana Smoothie

Ingredients
- 1 cup milk

- 1 1/2 bananas
- 5 (1 gram) packets low calorie granulated sugar substitute (such as Sweet 'n Low®)
- Add all ingredients to list

Directions

1. Blend milk, bananas, and sugar substitute in a blender or food processor until smooth.

Nutritional Information

- Calories: 280 kcal 14%
- Fat: 5.4 g 8%
- Carbs: 56.8g 18%
- Protein: 10 g 20%
- Cholesterol: 20 mg 7%
- Sodium: 102 mg 4%

Molasses Spice Smoothie

Ingredients

- 1 cup milk
- 1/2 cup oats
- 1/2 cup ice cubes
- 1 small frozen banana, sliced
- 2 tablespoons unsulfured molasses
- 1/2 teaspoon ground ginger
- 1/2 teaspoon ground cinnamon
- 1/4 teaspoon vanilla extract
- 1 pinch ground cloves
- Add all ingredients to list

Directions

1. Blend milk, oats, ice cubes, banana, molasses, ginger, cinnamon, vanilla extract, and cloves in a blender until smooth.

Nutritional Information

- Calories: 247 kcal 12%
- Fat: 4 g 6%
- Carbs: 47.1g 15%

- Protein: 7.3 g 15%
- Cholesterol: 10 mg 3%
- Sodium: 62 mg 2%

Moringa Coconut Smoothie

Ingredients
- 2 bananas
- 1 cup sliced frozen peaches
- 1/3 cup coconut milk
- 1 tablespoon moringa powder
- 1 tablespoon almond butter
- 1 cup water
- Add all ingredients to list

Directions
1. Layer bananas, peaches, coconut milk, moringa powder, and almond butter in a blender; add water. Blend mixture until very smooth, at least 1 minute.

Nutritional Information
- Calories: 252 kcal 13%
- Fat: 13.2 g 20%
- Carbs: 34.7g 11%
- Protein: 4 g 8%
- Cholesterol: 0 mg 0%
- Sodium: 48 mg 2%

Nectarine Sunshine Smoothie

Ingredients
- 2 large nectarines, pitted and quartered
- 1 banana, cut into pieces and frozen
- 1 large orange, peeled and quartered
- 1 cup vanilla yogurt
- 1 cup orange juice
- 1 tablespoon honey
- Add all ingredients to list

Directions

1. Place the nectarines, frozen banana chunks, orange, vanilla yogurt, orange juice, and honey into a blender, and blend until smooth.

Nutritional Information

- Calories: 184 kcal 9%
- Fat: 1.3 g 2%
- Carbs: 40.9g 13%
- Protein: 5.2 g 10%
- Cholesterol: 3 mg 1%
- Sodium: 42 mg 2%

Orange Banana Smoothie with Chia

Ingredients

- 1/3 cup vanilla-flavored or plain Greek yogurt
- 3 mandarin or clementine oranges - peeled, pith removed, sectioned
- 1/2 sliced, frozen banana
- 1 tablespoon truRoots® Organic Chia Seeds
- 3 ice cubes
- Add all ingredients to list

Directions

1. Place yogurt, oranges, banana, chia seeds and ice cubes in blender container. Cover and process until smooth.

Nutritional Information

- Calories: 334 kcal 17%
- Fat: 16.7 g 26%
- Carbs: 56.4g 18%
- Protein: 8.8 g 18%
- Cholesterol: 15 mg 5%
- Sodium: 53 mg 2%

Orange Banana Smoothie

"Filling enough to have as a breakfast - I recommend it!"
Serving: *5 m* | **Total Time:** *5 m*

Ingredients
- 1 cup cold milk
- 2 oranges, peeled and segmented
- 1 banana
- 1/4 cup sugar
- 1 pinch salt
- 1/2 (8 ounce) container vanilla fat-free yogurt
- 4 cubes ice
- Add all ingredients to list

Directions
1. In a blender, combine milk, oranges, banana, sugar, salt and yogurt. Blend for about 1 minute. Insert ice cubes, and blend until smooth. Pour into glasses and serve.

Nutritional Information
- Calories: 340 kcal 17%
- Fat: 2.9 g 4%
- Carbs: 73.7g 24%
- Protein: 9.1 g 18%
- Cholesterol: 11 mg 4%
- Sodium: 284 mg 11%

Orange Cream Drink

Ingredients
- 1 cup orange juice
- 1/2 cup apple juice
- 3 tablespoons honey
- 1/2 teaspoon vanilla extract
- 2 tablespoons nonfat dry milk powder
- 1 banana, sliced
- 2 cubes ice

- Add all ingredients to list

Directions

1. In a blender combine orange juice, apple juice, honey, vanilla, milk powder, banana and ice cubes. Blend on high speed for 30 seconds. Serve immediately.

Nutritional Information

- Calories: 263 kcal 13%
- Fat: 0.6 g < 1%
- Carbs: 63.6g 21%
- Protein: 4.3 g 9%
- Cholesterol: 1 mg < 1%
- Sodium: 45 mg 2%

Orange Sunrise Smoothie

Ingredients

- 1/2 cup orange juice
- 1 banana, frozen and chunked
- 1 peach, peeled and sliced
- 1/2 cup honeydew melon, cubed
- 1 (8 ounce) container orange yogurt
- 1 teaspoon white sugar
- 1/2 cup ice
- Add all ingredients to list

Directions

1. Combine the orange juice, banana, peach, honeydew melon, yogurt, sugar, and ice in a blender. Blend until smooth, or chunky, as desired. Pour into two glasses and serve.

Nutritional Information

- Calories: 239 kcal 12%
- Fat: 1.3 g 2%
- Carbs: 52g 17%
- Protein: 5.8 g 12%
- Cholesterol: 9 mg 3%
- Sodium: 69 mg 3%

Overnight Oats Blueberry Smoothie Bowl

Ingredients
- 1 cup rolled oats
- 1 1/4 cups unsweetened vanilla-flavored almond milk, divided
- 1 frozen banana, chopped
- 1 cup blueberries
- 1 teaspoon vanilla extract
- 1 teaspoon maple syrup, or to taste
- Topping:
- 2 tablespoons flaked coconut
- 1 tablespoon fresh blueberries
- 1 teaspoon chia seeds
- Add all ingredients to list

Directions
1. Combine oats and 2/3 cup almond milk in a bowl; refrigerate until oats have absorbed the liquid, 8 hours to overnight.
2. Combine oats-almond milk mixture, remaining almond milk, banana, 1 cup blueberries, vanilla extract, and maple syrup in a blender; blend until smooth.
3. Pour smoothie into 2 bowls and top with coconut, 1 tablespoon blueberries, and chia seeds.

Nutritional Information
- Calories: 354 kcal 18%
- Fat: 6.5 g 10%
- Carbs: 68.7g 22%
- Protein: 7.6 g 15%
- Cholesterol: 0 mg 0%
- Sodium: 118 mg 5%

Pacific Smoothie

Ingredients
- 10 ice cubes
- 1 banana
- 4 teaspoons maple syrup
- 4 teaspoons brown sugar
- 1 cup eggnog
- 1/4 cup orange juice

- 1/4 cup vanilla yogurt
- Add all ingredients to list

Directions
1. Blend the ice, banana, maple syrup, brown sugar, eggnog, orange juice, and vanilla yogurt together in a blender until smooth.

Nutritional Information
- Calories: 667 kcal 33%
- Fat: 20.3 g 31%
- Carbs: 112.1g 36%
- Protein: 14.4 g 29%
- Cholesterol: 153 mg 51%
- Sodium: 193 mg 8%

Papaya Surprise Smoothie

Ingredients
- 1 papaya - peeled, seeded and diced
- 1 banana, peeled and sliced
- 1/2 cup sliced fresh strawberries
- 1/3 cup milk
- 1/4 cup sugar
- 15 ice cubes
- Add all ingredients to list

Directions
1. In a blender, blend the papaya, banana, strawberries, milk, sugar, and ice cubes until smooth.

Nutritional Information
- Calories: 228 kcal 11%
- Fat: 1.3 g 2%
- Carbs: 55.1g 18%
- Protein: 2.9 g 6%
- Cholesterol: 3 mg 1%
- Sodium: 25 mg < 1%

PB Banana Oat Smoothie

Ingredients
- 1 banana, broken in half
- 1 cup ice
- 1/4 cup old-fashioned rolled oats
- 1/2 cup vanilla yogurt
- 1/2 cup skim milk
- 1 1/2 tablespoons peanut butter
- 1 teaspoon honey, or to taste
- 1 teaspoon ground cinnamon, or to taste
- Add all ingredients to list

Directions
1. Put banana, ice, oats, yogurt, skim milk, peanut butter, honey, and cinnamon, respectively, in a blender; blend until smooth.

Nutritional Information
- Calories: 499 kcal 25%
- Fat: 15.7 g 24%
- Carbs: 76.4g 25%
- Protein: 20.4 g 41%
- Cholesterol: 9 mg 3%
- Sodium: 255 mg 10%

PB&J Smoothie

Ingredients
- 2 cups almond milk
- 1 cup vanilla yogurt
- 1 banana
- 6 strawberries, hulled
- 1 tablespoon almond butter, or more to taste
- Add all ingredients to list

Directions
1. Combine almond milk, vanilla yogurt, banana, strawberries, and almond butter in a blender; blend until smooth.

Nutritional Information
- Calories: 577 kcal 29%
- Fat: 18.6 g 29%
- Carbs: 89.5g 29%
- Protein: 18.6 g 37%
- Cholesterol: 12 mg 4%
- Sodium: 556 mg 22%

PBnJ Workday Smoothie

Ingredients
- 20 frozen strawberries
- 1 frozen sliced banana
- 1/2 cup water, or as desired
- 1/4 cup vanilla fat-free yogurt
- 2 tablespoons creamy peanut butter
- Add all ingredients to list

Directions
1. Place strawberries, banana, water, and yogurt in a blender; blend until smooth, gradually adding more water if a thinner smoothie is desired. Add peanut butter blend until smooth.

Nutritional Information
- Calories: 426 kcal 21%
- Fat: 17.1 g 26%
- Carbs: 63.4g 20%
- Protein: 13.5 g 27%
- Cholesterol: < 1 mg < 1%
- Sodium: 200 mg 8%

Peach Banana Smoothie

Ingredients
- 1 cup plain yogurt
- 1 (15.25 ounce) can peaches
- 2 bananas, sliced
- 1/4 cup orange juice

- 1/4 cup white sugar, or to taste
- 2 cubes ice
- Add all ingredients to list

Directions

1. Blend yogurt, peaches, bananas, orange juice, sugar, and ice in a blender on high until the ice is crushed and the smoothie is to your desired consistency.

Nutritional Information

- Calories: 194 kcal 10%
- Fat: 1.2 g 2%
- Carbs: 44.4g 14%
- Protein: 4.6 g 9%
- Cholesterol: 4 mg 1%
- Sodium: 48 mg 2%

Peaches 'N Cream Banana Breakfast Smoothie

Ingredients

- 1 1/4 cups milk
- 1/4 cup vanilla yogurt
- 1 banana, broken into chunks
- 1 packet peaches and cream flavor instant oatmeal
- 2 packets granular no-calorie sucralose sweetener (such as Splenda®) (optional)
- 5 ice cubes
- Add all ingredients to list

Directions

1. Place the milk, yogurt, banana, instant oatmeal, sweetener, and ice cubes into a blender. Cover, and puree until smooth. Pour into glasses to serve.

Nutritional Information

- Calories: 223 kcal 11%
- Fat: 4.8 g 7%
- Carbs: 39.2g 13%
- Protein: 8.7 g 17%
- Cholesterol: 14 mg 5%
- Sodium: 180 mg 7%

Peanut Butter and Banana Smoothie

"Like a peanut butter and banana sandwich in liquid form. Makes a nice thick breakfast smoothie."
***Serving:** 10 m | **Total Time:** 10 m*

Ingredients
- 1 banana
- 1/8 cup peanut butter
- 1/2 cup soy milk
- 2 tablespoons honey
- Add all ingredients to list

Directions
1. In a blender, combine banana, peanut butter and soy milk. Blend until smooth. Pour into glasses and drizzle with honey for garnish.

Nutritional Information
- Calories: 488 kcal 24%
- Fat: 18.8 g 29%
- Carbs: 75.5g 24%
- Protein: 13.5 g 27%
- Cholesterol: 0 mg 0%
- Sodium: 213 mg 9%

Peanut Butter and Jelly Smoothie

Ingredients
- 2 cups milk
- 2 tablespoons blackberry jelly
- 2 tablespoons peanut butter
- 1 bananas, frozen and chunked
- 2 tablespoons honey
- 2 teaspoons wheat germ
- Add all ingredients to list

Directions
1. In a blender combine milk, jelly, peanut butter, banana, honey and wheat germ. Blend until smooth.

Nutritional Information
- Calories: 157 kcal 8%
- Fat: 5.4 g 8%
- Carbs: 23.9g 8%
- Protein: 5.4 g 11%
- Cholesterol: 8 mg 3%
- Sodium: 71 mg 3%

Peanut Butter Banana Boost Smoothie

Ingredients
- 1/2 cup skim milk
- 1/2 cup plain low fat Greek-style yogurt
- 2 tablespoons KRAFT All Natural Peanut Butter
- 1 tablespoon oats
- 1 tablespoon honey
- 1 small banana, sliced
- 4 ice cubes
- Add all ingredients to list

Directions
1. Blend all ingredients except ice in blender until smooth.
2. Add ice; blend until thickened.
3. Serve immediately.

Nutritional Information
- Calories: 469 kcal 23%
- Fat: 17 g 26%
- Carbs: 56.4g 18%
- Protein: 23.6 g 47%
- Cholesterol: 8 mg 3%
- Sodium: 93 mg 4%

Peanut Butter Banana Breakfast Smoothie

Ingredients
- 2 frozen bananas (peel before you freeze)
- 2 cups almond milk
- 2 cups ice cubes
- 1/2 cup chunky peanut butter
- 2 tablespoons wheat germ
- 2 tablespoons ground flax seed
- 1 tablespoon honey
- Add all ingredients to list

Directions
1. Blend bananas, almond milk, ice, peanut butter, wheat germ, flax seed, and honey in a blender until smooth.

Nutritional Information
- Calories: 335 kcal 17%
- Fat: 20.5 g 32%
- Carbs: 32.6g 11%
- Protein: 10.9 g 22%
- Cholesterol: 0 mg 0%
- Sodium: 243 mg 10%

Peanut Butter Banana Smoothie

"It is so refreshing and it's sweet and tasty."
Serving: 5 m | Total Time: 5 m

Ingredients
- 2 bananas, broken into chunks
- 2 cups milk
- 1/2 cup peanut butter
- 2 tablespoons honey, or to taste
- 2 cups ice cubes
- Add all ingredients to list

Directions

1. Place bananas, milk, peanut butter, honey, and ice cubes in a blender; blend until smooth, about 30 seconds.

Nutritional Information

- Calories: 335 kcal 17%
- Fat: 18.8 g 29%
- Carbs: 34.1g 11%
- Protein: 12.8 g 26%
- Cholesterol: 10 mg 3%
- Sodium: 203 mg 8%

Peanut Butter Mango Smoothie

Ingredients

- 1 cup vanilla yogurt
- 1 banana, broken into chunks
- 1/2 cup frozen mango chunks
- 2 tablespoons peanut butter, or to taste
- Add all ingredients to list

Directions

1. Blend yogurt, banana, mango, and peanut butter together in a blender until smooth.

Nutritional Information

- Calories: 279 kcal 14%
- Fat: 10 g 15%
- Carbs: 40.6g 13%
- Protein: 11 g 22%
- Cholesterol: 6 mg 2%
- Sodium: 157 mg 6%

Penny's Smoothie

Ingredients

- 1 banana
- 1/4 cup frozen blueberries

- 3/4 cup frozen peach slices
- 1/4 cup yogurt
- 2 tablespoons all fruit blueberry syrup
- 1/8 cup rice milk
- Add all ingredients to list

Directions
1. In a blender, combine banana, frozen blueberries, frozen peach slices, yogurt and syrup. Blend until smooth. add rice milk and blend to desired consistency. Pour into glasses and serve.

Nutritional Information
- Calories: 139 kcal 7%
- Fat: 0.7 g 1%
- Carbs: 33.1g 11%
- Protein: 2.1 g 4%
- Cholesterol: 1 mg < 1%
- Sodium: 24 mg < 1%

Perfect Peach Smoothie

Ingredients
- 1 large peach, sliced and frozen
- 1 banana, cut into pieces and frozen
- 1/2 cup orange juice
- 1/2 cup soy milk
- 1 tablespoon ground flax seed (optional)
- Add all ingredients to list

Directions
1. Blend peach, banana, orange juice, soy milk, and flax seed in a blender until smooth.

Nutritional Information
- Calories: 297 kcal 15%
- Fat: 5.7 g 9%
- Carbs: 57.5g 19%
- Protein: 7.4 g 15%
- Cholesterol: 0 mg 0%

- Sodium: 72 mg 3%

Persimmon Green Smoothie

Ingredients
- 1 1/2 cups almond milk
- 1/3 cup plain kefir
- 1 1/3 cups chopped kale, or as needed
- 1 1/3 cups chopped fresh spinach, or as needed
- 1 1/3 cups chopped Swiss chard, or as needed
- 3 persimmons, peeled
- 1 1/2 frozen bananas
- 1/2 avocado, peeled and pitted
- 1 tablespoon chia seeds
- 1 teaspoon honey, or more to taste (optional)
- Add all ingredients to list

Directions
1. Blend almond milk and kefir together in a blender; add kale, spinach, and Swiss chard. Blend until smooth and the mixture reaches the 4 cup mark. Add persimmons, bananas, avocado, chia seeds, and honey; puree until smooth.

Nutritional Information
- Calories: 172 kcal 9%
- Fat: 6.4 g 10%
- Carbs: 28.3g 9%
- Protein: 3.9 g 8%
- Cholesterol: 0 mg 0%
- Sodium: 120 mg 5%

Pina Colada Smoothie Vegan

Ingredients
- 3 cubes ice cubes, or as needed
- 1 banana
- 1 cup fresh pineapple chunks
- 1/2 cup coconut milk
- 1/2 cup soy milk

- 1 tablespoon agave nectar
- 1 tablespoon ground flax seed
- 1 teaspoon pure vanilla extract
- Add all ingredients to list

Directions
1. Blend ice, banana, pineapple, coconut milk, soy milk, agave nectar, flax seed, and vanilla extract in a blender until smooth. Pour smoothie into a tall glass.

Nutritional Information
- Calories: 586 kcal 29%
- Fat: 29.8 g 46%
- Carbs: 78g 25%
- Protein: 9.7 g 19%
- Cholesterol: 0 mg 0%
- Sodium: 84 mg 3%

Pineapple and Banana Smoothie

"A gorgeous and indulgent smoothie, but totally healthy!"
***Serving:** 3 m | **Total Time:** 3 m*

Ingredients
- 4 ice cubes
- 1/4 fresh pineapple - peeled, cored and cubed
- 1 large banana, cut into chunks
- 1 cup pineapple or apple juice
- Add all ingredients to list

Directions
1. Place ice cubes, pineapple, banana, and pineapple juice into the bowl of a blender. Puree on high until smooth.

Nutritional Information
- Calories: 313 kcal 16%
- Fat: 0.9 g 1%
- Carbs: 78.7g 25%
- Protein: 3 g 6%
- Cholesterol: 0 mg 0%

- Sodium: 10 mg < 1%

Pineapple Banana Smoothie

Ingredients
- 1/2 cup whole seedless grapes
- 1 1/2 cups apple juice
- 1 1/2 cups plain kefir (cultured milk)
- 1 large banana
- 1 1/2 cups frozen pineapple chunks
- 1/3 cup chopped pitted dates (such as Sun-Maid®)
- Add all ingredients to list

Directions
1. Combine grapes, apple juice, kefir, banana, pineapple, and dates, in this order, in a blender; blend until smooth.

Nutritional Information
- Calories: 419 kcal 21%
- Fat: 7 g 11%
- Carbs: 87.4g 28%
- Protein: 8.2 g 16%
- Cholesterol: 0 mg 0%
- Sodium: 89 mg 4%

Pineapple Carrot Smoothie

Ingredients
- 1 frozen banana, broken into chunks
- 1 cup frozen pineapple chunks
- 1 carrot, cut into chunks
- 1 tablespoon hemp seeds
- 1/2 teaspoon finely grated ginger
- 1/4 teaspoon finely grated orange zest
- 1 pinch ground cinnamon
- 1/2 cup coconut milk
- 1/2 cup water

- Add all ingredients to list

Directions

1. Place banana, pineapple, carrot, hemp seeds, ginger, orange zest, cinnamon, coconut milk, and water in a blender in the order listed; blend on high until creamy and smooth.

Nutritional Information

- Calories: 247 kcal 12%
- Fat: 14.6 g 23%
- Carbs: 30g 10%
- Protein: 4.2 g 8%
- Cholesterol: 0 mg 0%
- Sodium: 32 mg 1%

Pineapple Creamsicle® Smoothie

Ingredients

- 1/2 fresh pineapple - peeled, cored, and chopped
- 1 cup vanilla yogurt
- 1 banana, cut into chunks
- 1/2 cup orange juice
- 32 ice cubes, or as needed
- Add all ingredients to list

Directions

1. Blend pineapple, yogurt, banana, and orange juice together in a blender until smooth. Add ice and blend until ice is completely crushed and incorporated.

Nutritional Information

- Calories: 122 kcal 6%
- Fat: 1 g 2%
- Carbs: 26.2g 8%
- Protein: 3.9 g 8%
- Cholesterol: 3 mg 1%
- Sodium: 47 mg 2%

Pineapple Delight Smoothie

Ingredients
- 2 cups milk
- 2 bananas, frozen and chunked
- 6 pineapple rings
- 1 tablespoon honey
- Add all ingredients to list

Directions
1. In a blender combine milk, frozen bananas, pineapple and honey. Blend until smooth.

Nutritional Information
- Calories: 197 kcal 10%
- Fat: 2.6 g 4%
- Carbs: 40.8g 13%
- Protein: 4.7 g 9%
- Cholesterol: 10 mg 3%
- Sodium: 58 mg 2%

Pineapple Jupiter

Ingredients
- 2/3 cup cold milk
- 1/3 cup cold water
- 1 (6 ounce) can frozen pineapple juice concentrate
- 1 tablespoon white sugar
- 1/2 teaspoon vanilla extract
- 1 banana, peeled and chopped
- 6 ice cubes
- ground cinnamon to taste
- Add all ingredients to list

Directions
1. In a blender, blend the milk, water, pineapple juice concentrate, sugar, vanilla extract, banana, and ice cubes until smooth. Sprinkle with cinnamon, and serve immediately.

Nutritional Information

- Calories: 315 kcal 16%
- Fat: 1.9 g 3%
- Carbs: 71.9g 23%
- Protein: 4.8 g 10%
- Cholesterol: 7 mg 2%
- Sodium: 40 mg 2%

Power 9 Protein Smoothie

Ingredients

- 1 cup soy milk
- 1 large frozen banana
- 1 tablespoon plain yogurt
- 1 tablespoon peanut butter
- 1 tablespoon tahini
- 1 tablespoon flax seed meal
- 1 tablespoon almond flour
- 1 tablespoon wheat germ
- 1 scoop protein powder
- Add all ingredients to list

Directions

1. Blend soy milk, banana, yogurt, peanut butter, and tahini together in a blender. Add flax seed meal, almond flour, wheat germ, and protein powder; blend to combine.

Nutritional Information

- Calories: 664 kcal 33%
- Fat: 29.7 g 46%
- Carbs: 69g 22%
- Protein: 37.2 g 74%
- Cholesterol: < 1 mg < 1%
- Sodium: 414 mg 17%

Power Drink ***THE ORANGE***

Ingredients
- 2 ripe bananas, peeled
- 4 carrots, scrubbed and trimmed
- 2 apples, cored
- 1 (8 ounce) container plain yogurt
- 1/2 cup orange juice
- 1 lemon, juiced
- 1 tablespoon ground flax seed
- 1 pinch salt
- 4 pitted dates, or to taste (optional)
- 8 cubes ice, or as needed (optional)
- Add all ingredients to list

Directions
1. Blend the bananas, carrots, apples, yogurt, orange juice, lemon juice, flax seed, salt, dates, and ice cubes in a blender until smooth.

Nutritional Information
- Calories: 204 kcal 10%
- Fat: 2.2 g 3%
- Carbs: 44.9g 14%
- Protein: 5.2 g 10%
- Cholesterol: 3 mg 1%
- Sodium: 85 mg 3%

Power Packed Smoothie

Ingredients
- 1 cup cold water
- 1 small banana
- 1/2 cup spinach, or more to taste
- 1 teaspoon spirulina powder
- Add all ingredients to list

Directions
1. Place cold water, banana, and spinach leaves in a blender; blend to combine, about 5 seconds. Add spirulina powder and blend until smooth, 1 minute

more.

Nutritional Information
- Calories: 100 kcal 5%
- Fat: 0.6 g < 1%
- Carbs: 24.2g 8%
- Protein: 2.9 g 6%
- Cholesterol: 0 mg 0%
- Sodium: 44 mg 2%

Prairie Berry Smoothie

Ingredients
- 3/4 cup milk
- 1/4 cup frozen blueberries
- 1/4 cup frozen raspberries
- 1/4 cup frozen mango chunks
- 2 tablespoons vanilla yogurt, or more to taste
- 1 banana
- Add all ingredients to list

Directions
1. Blend milk, blueberries, raspberries, mango, and yogurt together in a blender until smooth. Add banana and blend until smooth.

Nutritional Information
- Calories: 338 kcal 17%
- Fat: 4.8 g 7%
- Carbs: 69g 22%
- Protein: 9.9 g 20%
- Cholesterol: 16 mg 5%
- Sodium: 98 mg 4%

Pre Packaged Smoothies

Ingredients
- 4 (8 ounce) containers plain lowfat yogurt
- 2 cups sliced fresh strawberries

- 2 cups fresh blueberries
- 2 bananas, halved
- Add all ingredients to list

Directions

1. Transfer each container of yogurt into a muffin cup and freeze solid, about 4 hours. Remove frozen yogurt; place 1 portion of frozen yogurt into a resealable plastic bag and add 1/2 cup strawberries, 1/2 cup blueberries, and half a banana to each bag. Store the bags in the freezer until serving time. Place contents of a bag into a blender and blend until smooth.

Nutritional Information

- Calories: 263 kcal 13%
- Fat: 4.2 g 6%
- Carbs: 46.3g 15%
- Protein: 13.7 g 27%
- Cholesterol: 14 mg 5%
- Sodium: 161 mg 6%

Pretend You're in the Tropics Smoothie

Ingredients

- 1 banana, sliced
- 1 mango - peeled, seeded, and diced
- 1 (6 ounce) container coconut yogurt
- 6 fluid ounces 1% milk
- 1 tablespoon ground flax seed
- Add all ingredients to list

Directions

1. Blend banana, mango, coconut yogurt, milk, and ground flax seed in a blender until smooth.

Nutritional Information

- Calories: 219 kcal 11%
- Fat: 6.1 g 9%
- Carbs: 40.8g 13%
- Protein: 4.8 g 10%
- Cholesterol: 4 mg 1%
- Sodium: 55 mg 2%

Protein Packed Spinach Smoothie

Ingredients
- 2 cups fresh spinach leaves
- 2 bananas, cut into chunks
- 1 ounce firm tofu
- 2 tablespoons unsweetened shredded coconut
- 1/2 cup frozen peach slices
- 1/2 cup frozen pineapple chunks
- 1/2 cup frozen mango chunks
- 1/2 cup frozen strawberries
- 1 cup unsweetened apple juice, or to taste
- Add all ingredients to list

Directions
1. Place spinach, bananas, tofu, coconut, peaches, pineapple, mango, and strawberries, respectively, in a blender; pour in apple juice. Blend until desired consistency is reached, adding more apple juice as necessary.

Nutritional Information
- Calories: 377 kcal 19%
- Fat: 5.4 g 8%
- Carbs: 84.8g 27%
- Protein: 4.8 g 10%
- Cholesterol: 0 mg 0%
- Sodium: 39 mg 2%

Pumpkin Apple Smoothie

Ingredients
- 1 1/2 cups almond milk
- 1 apple, cored and chopped
- 1/2 sliced frozen banana
- 1/4 cup frozen pumpkin puree
- 3 dates, pitted
- 3 cubes ice (optional)
- 2 tablespoons ground chia seeds
- 2 tablespoons large flake oats

- 1 tablespoon hemp seeds
- 1 1/2 teaspoons pumpkin pie spice
- 1 teaspoon molasses
- 1 teaspoon honey (optional)
- 1/4 teaspoon pure vanilla extract
- Add all ingredients to list

Directions

1. Blend almond milk, apple, banana, pumpkin puree, dates, ice, chia seeds, oats, hemp seeds, pumpkin pie spice, molasses, honey, and vanilla extract in a blender until smooth.

Nutritional Information

- Calories: 534 kcal 27%
- Fat: 14.7 g 23%
- Carbs: 96.9g 31%
- Protein: 11 g 22%
- Cholesterol: 0 mg 0%
- Sodium: 399 mg 16%

Pumpkin Banana Smoothie

Ingredients

- 1 cup pumpkin puree
- 1 cup milk
- 1 banana, sliced
- 2 tablespoons brown sugar
- 1/4 teaspoon ground cinnamon
- 1/4 teaspoon vanilla extract
- Add all ingredients to list

Directions

1. Spoon pumpkin puree into a resealable bag and freeze, 8 hours to overnight.
2. Remove pumpkin from freezer and allow to soften at room temperature, 5 to 10 minutes.
3. Pour milk into the blender; add pumpkin, banana, brown sugar, cinnamon, and vanilla extract. Blend until smooth, about 3 minutes.

Nutritional Information

- Calories: 209 kcal 10%

- Fat: 2.9 g 5%
- Carbs: 42.7g 14%
- Protein: 6 g 12%
- Cholesterol: 10 mg 3%
- Sodium: 350 mg 14%

Pumpkin Banana Tofu Smoothie

Ingredients
- 1 banana
- 1 cup milk
- 1 cup pumpkin puree
- 1/2 cup tofu
- 6 almonds, or more to taste
- 1 tablespoon ground cinnamon
- 1 teaspoon ground nutmeg
- Add all ingredients to list

Directions
1. Blend banana, milk, pumpkin, tofu, almonds, cinnamon, and nutmeg together in a blender until smooth.

Nutritional Information
- Calories: 239 kcal 12%
- Fat: 8.3 g 13%
- Carbs: 34.5g 11%
- Protein: 12 g 24%
- Cholesterol: 10 mg 3%
- Sodium: 351 mg 14%

Pumpkin Peanut Butter Smoothie

Ingredients
- 1 banana, broken into chunks
- 3 whole frozen strawberries, or more to taste
- 3/4 cup milk
- 1/2 cup plain yogurt
- 1/4 cup pumpkin puree

- 2 tablespoons creamy peanut butter
- 1 tablespoon brown sugar
- 1/4 teaspoon ground cinnamon
- 1 pinch ground nutmeg
- 8 ice cubes, or as desired
- 1/4 cup whipped cream, or more to taste (optional)
- 1 pinch ground cinnamon (optional)
- Add all ingredients to list

Directions

1. Blend banana, strawberries, milk, yogurt, pumpkin puree, peanut butter, brown sugar, 1/4 teaspoon cinnamon, and nutmeg in a blender until smooth; add ice cubes and again blend until smooth. Pour smoothie into 4 glasses and top with whipped cream and a pinch of cinnamon.

Nutritional Information

- Calories: 149 kcal 7%
- Fat: 6.6 g 10%
- Carbs: 18.8g 6%
- Protein: 5.8 g 12%
- Cholesterol: 8 mg 3%
- Sodium: 122 mg 5%

Pumpkin Pie Smoothie for 2

Ingredients

- 8 ice cubes, or as desired
- 1 banana
- 1/4 cup yogurt
- 1/4 cup pumpkin puree
- 1/8 teaspoon ground cinnamon
- 1 pinch ground ginger
- Add all ingredients to list

Directions

1. Blend ice cubes, banana, yogurt, pumpkin, cinnamon, and ginger together in a blender until smooth.

Nutritional Information

- Calories: 84 kcal 4%

- Fat: 0.8 g 1%
- Carbs: 18.6g 6%
- Protein: 2.6 g 5%
- Cholesterol: 2 mg < 1%
- Sodium: 99 mg 4%

Pumpkin Shake

Ingredients
- 4 cubes ice, or more if desired
- 1 cup skim milk
- 1/3 cup pumpkin puree
- 1/3 cup plain fat-free Greek yogurt
- 1/2 frozen banana, cut into chunks
- 1 pinch ground cinnamon
- 1 pinch ground ginger
- 1 pinch ground nutmeg
- 1 pinch ground allspice
- 1 teaspoon vanilla extract
- Add all ingredients to list

Directions
1. Blend ice, milk, pumpkin puree, yogurt, banana, cinnamon, ginger, nutmeg, allspice, and vanilla in a blender until smooth.

Nutritional Information
- Calories: 230 kcal 12%
- Fat: 1.1 g 2%
- Carbs: 38.5g 12%
- Protein: 16.6 g 33%
- Cholesterol: 5 mg 2%
- Sodium: 332 mg 13%

Pumpkin Spice Protein Drink

Ingredients
- 1 cup unsweetened almond milk
- 2 bananas, sliced and frozen

- 1/2 cup canned pumpkin
- 2 dates, pitted
- 1 scoop vanilla protein powder
- 1/2 teaspoon vanilla extract
- 1 pinch ground nutmeg
- 1 pinch ground cinnamon
- 1 pinch ground cloves
- 1 pinch ground ginger
- Add all ingredients to list

Directions

1. Blend almond milk, bananas, pumpkin, dates, protein powder, vanilla extract, nutmeg, cinnamon, cloves, and ginger together in a blender until smooth.

Nutritional Information

- Calories: 280 kcal 14%
- Fat: 3 g 5%
- Carbs: 45.6g 15%
- Protein: 22 g 44%
- Cholesterol: 6 mg 2%
- Sodium: 192 mg 8%

Purple Monstrosity Fruit Smoothie

"This is a great smoothie for breakfast - and sometimes dinner! You can substitute the orange juice with any mix of juices or even soy milk! The soy milk adds more of a milk shake quality than the juice does."
***Serving:** 5 m | **Total Time:** 5 m*

Ingredients

- 2 frozen bananas, skins removed and cut in chunks
- 1/2 cup frozen blueberries
- 1 cup orange juice
- 1 tablespoon honey (optional)
- 1 teaspoon vanilla extract (optional)
- Add all ingredients to list

Directions

1. Place bananas, blueberries and juice in a blender, puree. Use honey and/or vanilla to taste. Use more or less liquid depending on the thickness you want

for your smoothie.

Nutritional Information
- Calories: 87 kcal 4%
- Fat: 0.4 g < 1%
- Carbs: 21.4g 7%
- Protein: 0.9 g 2%
- Cholesterol: 0 mg 0%
- Sodium: 1 mg < 1%

Purple Moose Canadian Smoothie

Ingredients
- 15 ice cubes
- 1 ripe banana
- 1/2 cup vanilla rice milk
- 1/4 cup fresh blueberries
- 2 tablespoons natural peanut butter
- 2 tablespoons maple syrup
- Add all ingredients to list

Directions
1. Combine ice cubes, banana, rice milk, blueberries, peanut butter, and maple syrup in a blender; blend on low speed. Increase speed to medium-high and blend until smooth.

Nutritional Information
- Calories: 241 kcal 12%
- Fat: 8.7 g 13%
- Carbs: 39.9g 13%
- Protein: 4.9 g 10%
- Cholesterol: 0 mg 0%
- Sodium: 70 mg 3%

Purple Power Punch Smoothie My Kids' Fave

Ingredients
- 1/2 cup nonfat vanilla yogurt (such as Dannon® Light and Fit®)

- 1/2 cup sliced strawberries
- 1/2 cup water
- 1/2 cup nonfat powdered milk
- 1 banana, cut in chunks
- 1/4 cup blueberries, or to taste
- 1/4 cup raspberries, or to taste
- 1/4 cup blackberries, or to taste
- 2 scoops vanilla whey protein powder
- 1 cup crushed ice
- 3 tablespoons turbinado sugar (such as Sugar in the Raw®)
- 1 tablespoon honey
- Add all ingredients to list

Directions

1. Pulse yogurt, strawberries, water, powdered milk, banana, blueberries, raspberries, blackberries, and protein powder together in a blender until well-mixed. Add ice, sugar, and honey and blend until smooth.

Nutritional Information

- Calories: 177 kcal 9%
- Fat: 0.7 g 1%
- Carbs: 26.5g 9%
- Protein: 17.7 g 35%
- Cholesterol: 6 mg 2%
- Sodium: 142 mg 6%

Quick Avocado Smoothie

Ingredients

- 1 1/4 cups almond milk
- 1 avocado - peeled, pitted, and sliced
- 1 small banana, sliced
- 1/4 cup ice, or as needed
- 1 tablespoon honey (optional)
- Add all ingredients to list

Directions

1. Blend almond milk, avocado, banana, ice, and honey in a blender until smooth.

Nutritional Information
- Calories: 555 kcal 28%
- Fat: 33.1 g 51%
- Carbs: 68.2g 22%
- Protein: 6.5 g 13%
- Cholesterol: 0 mg 0%
- Sodium: 218 mg 9%

Quick Green Smoothie

Ingredients
- 1 cup stemmed kale
- 1 cup skim milk
- 1 sliced frozen banana
- 1/2 green apple, cut into chunks
- 1/2 pear, cut into chunks
- 1/4 cup old-fashioned rolled oats
- 1 tablespoon peanut butter
- 1 tablespoon flax seed meal
- 1 tablespoon wheat germ
- 2 sprigs fresh parsley, or more to taste
- Add all ingredients to list

Directions
1. Blend kale, milk, banana, apple, pear, oats, peanut butter, flax seed meal, wheat germ, and parsley in a blender until smooth.

Nutritional Information
- Calories: 561 kcal 28%
- Fat: 14.9 g 23%
- Carbs: 94.3g 30%
- Protein: 23.6 g 47%
- Cholesterol: 5 mg 2%
- Sodium: 245 mg 10%

Quick Kale and Banana Smoothie

Ingredients
- 2 cups chopped kale
- 1 banana, cut into chunks
- 1/2 cup coconut milk
- 1/2 cup frozen strawberries, or more to taste
- Add all ingredients to list

Directions
1. Blend kale, banana, coconut milk, and strawberries together in a blender until smooth.

Nutritional Information
- Calories: 433 kcal 22%
- Fat: 25.6 g 39%
- Carbs: 53.6g 17%
- Protein: 8.5 g 17%
- Cholesterol: 0 mg 0%
- Sodium: 76 mg 3%

Quick Kale and Turmeric Smoothie

Ingredients
- 6 ice cubes
- 1 cup almond milk
- 1 banana
- 3 leaves kale, large stems discarded, leaves chopped
- 1/4 cup flax seed meal
- 2 tablespoons chopped fresh ginger
- 2 tablespoons chopped fresh turmeric root
- 1 tablespoon almond butter
- 1/4 teaspoon stevia
- 1/4 teaspoon cayenne pepper
- 1/8 teaspoon ground black pepper
- Add all ingredients to list

Directions
1. Blend ice cubes, almond milk, banana, kale, flax seed meal, ginger, turmeric root, almond butter, stevia powder, cayenne pepper, and ground black pepper together in a blender until smooth.

Nutritional Information
- Calories: 471 kcal 24%
- Fat: 25 g 38%
- Carbs: 58.1g 19%
- Protein: 12.4 g 25%
- Cholesterol: 0 mg 0%
- Sodium: 274 mg 11%

Quick Start Breakfast Drink

Ingredients
- 2 cups pineapple juice
- 2 bananas
- 2 cups vanilla yogurt
- 1 cup strawberries, hulled
- 1/4 cup wheat germ
- 1 teaspoon vanilla extract
- Add all ingredients to list

Directions
1. In a blender combine pineapple juice, bananas yogurt, strawberries, wheat germ and vanilla extract. Blend until smooth.

Nutritional Information
- Calories: 263 kcal 13%
- Fat: 2.7 g 4%
- Carbs: 53.1g 17%
- Protein: 9 g 18%
- Cholesterol: 6 mg 2%
- Sodium: 85 mg 3%

Quick Strawberry Oatmeal Breakfast Smoothie

Ingredients
- 1/2 cup rolled oats
- 1 teaspoon chia seeds
- 14 frozen strawberries
- 6 ounces nonfat vanilla Greek yogurt
- 1 banana, broken into chunks
- 1/2 cup almond milk
- 1/2 teaspoon vanilla extract
- Add all ingredients to list

Directions
1. Blend oats and chia seeds together in a blender to a fine consistency. Add strawberries, yogurt, banana, almond milk, and vanilla extract; blend until smooth.

Nutritional Information
- Calories: 245 kcal 12%
- Fat: 2.6 g 4%
- Carbs: 45.8g 15%
- Protein: 11.1 g 22%
- Cholesterol: 5 mg 2%
- Sodium: 84 mg 3%

Rainier Cherry Berry Smoothie

Ingredients
- 1 banana
- 3/4 cup blueberries
- 1/2 cup fat-free vanilla yogurt
- 6 large fresh strawberries, halved
- 12 Rainier cherries, pitted and halved
- 1/4 cup fat-free milk
- Add all ingredients to list

Directions

1. Combine banana, blueberries, vanilla yogurt, strawberries, cherries, and milk in a blender; blend until smooth, about 60 seconds.

Nutritional Information

- Calories: 199 kcal 10%
- Fat: 1.1 g 2%
- Carbs: 44.7g 14%
- Protein: 6.3 g 13%
- Cholesterol: 2 mg < 1%
- Sodium: 62 mg 2%

Raspberry Banana Tofu Shake

Ingredients

- 1 (12 ounce) package firm silken tofu
- 1 cup fat free soy milk
- 1 banana
- 1 cup raspberries
- 1/4 cup frozen orange juice concentrate
- Add all ingredients to list

Directions

1. In a blender, mix tofu, soy milk, banana, raspberries, and orange juice concentrate. Blend until smooth.

Nutritional Information

- Calories: 149 kcal 7%
- Fat: 2.6 g 4%
- Carbs: 24.6g 8%
- Protein: 8.3 g 17%
- Cholesterol: 0 mg 0%
- Sodium: 46 mg 2%

Raspberry Blackberry Smoothie

Ingredients

- 1 small banana

- 1/2 cup blackberries
- 1 cup fresh raspberries
- 1 (6 ounce) container vanilla yogurt
- 1 tablespoon honey
- 4 ice cubes
- Add all ingredients to list

Directions
1. Place banana, blackberries, raspberries, yogurt, honey, and ice cubes into a blender. Blend until smooth.

Nutritional Information
- Calories: 195 kcal 10%
- Fat: 1.7 g 3%
- Carbs: 42.5g 14%
- Protein: 5.8 g 12%
- Cholesterol: 4 mg 1%
- Sodium: 59 mg 2%

Raspberry Chocolate Smoothie

Ingredients
- 3/4 cup chocolate flavored soy milk
- 3/4 cup chocolate sorbet
- 1 1/4 cups frozen unsweetened raspberries
- 1/2 banana, peeled and sliced
- 1 leaf fresh mint, chopped
- Add all ingredients to list

Directions
1. In a blender, blend the soy milk, sorbet, raspberries, and banana until smooth. Garnish with mint to serve.

Nutritional Information
- Calories: 341 kcal 17%
- Fat: 1.8 g 3%
- Carbs: 78.7g 25%
- Protein: 5.5 g 11%
- Cholesterol: 0 mg 0%

- Sodium: 90 mg 4%

Raspberry OJ Banana Smoothie

Ingredients
- 1 1/2 cups ice cubes
- 1 cup fresh raspberries
- 1 cup orange juice
- 1 banana, cut into chunks
- 1/2 cup vanilla fat-free yogurt
- 1 teaspoon honey, or to taste
- Add all ingredients to list

Directions
1. Blend ice cubes, raspberries, orange juice, banana, yogurt, and honey in a blender until smooth.

Nutritional Information
- Calories: 206 kcal 10%
- Fat: 0.9 g 1%
- Carbs: 47.3g 15%
- Protein: 5.2 g 10%
- Cholesterol: < 1 mg < 1%
- Sodium: 49 mg 2%

Raw Mango Monster Smoothie

Ingredients
- 1 tablespoon flax seeds
- 2 tablespoons pepitas (raw pumpkin seeds)
- 1 ripe mango, cubed
- 1 frozen banana, quartered
- 1/3 cup water, or more to taste
- 3 ice cubes
- 2 leaves kale, or more to taste
- Add all ingredients to list

Directions

1. Blend flax seeds in a blender until finely ground; add pepitas and blend until ground, about 1 minute.
2. Place mango, banana, water, ice cubes, and kale in the blender; blend until smooth, kale is fully incorporated, and the smoothie is uniform in color, about 3 minutes. Thin with more water to reach desired consistency.

Nutritional Information

*   Calories: 381 kcal 19%
*   Fat: 14.1 g 22%
*   Carbs: 63g 20%
*   Protein: 9.8 g 20%
*   Cholesterol: 0 mg 0%
*   Sodium: 32 mg 1%

Raw Super Food Oat Smoothie

Ingredients

*   2 sweet apples, chopped
*   2 cups almond milk
*   2 bananas
*   1 tablespoon almond butter
*   1 tablespoon coconut sugar
*   1 tablespoon maca powder
*   1 teaspoon spirulina powder
*   1 teaspoon chlorella powder
*   1 1/2 cups oats
*   Add all ingredients to list

Directions

1. Place apples and almond milk in a blender; blend until smooth. Add bananas and blend. Add almond butter, coconut sugar, maca powder, spirulina powder, and chlorella powder and blend until smooth. Add oats and blend until smooth.

Nutritional Information

*   Calories: 195 kcal 10%
*   Fat: 4.1 g 6%
*   Carbs: 36.9g 12%
*   Protein: 4.7 g 9%

- Cholesterol: 0 mg 0%
- Sodium: 72 mg 3%

Razzy Blue Smoothie

Ingredients
- 1 banana
- 16 whole almonds
- 1/4 cup rolled oats
- 1 tablespoon flaxseed meal
- 1 cup frozen blueberries
- 1 cup raspberry yogurt
- 1/4 cup Concord grape juice
- 1 cup 1% buttermilk
- Add all ingredients to list

Directions
1. Peel the banana and cut into 1/2-inch chunks. Chill in freezer until solid, about 2 hours.
2. Place the almonds, oats, and flaxseed meal into a blender; pulse until finely ground. Add the frozen banana, frozen blueberries, yogurt, grape juice, and buttermilk; puree until smooth.

Nutritional Information
- Calories: 262 kcal 13%
- Fat: 6.5 g 10%
- Carbs: 44.5g 14%
- Protein: 8.8 g 18%
- Cholesterol: 8 mg 3%
- Sodium: 142 mg 6%

Red White and Blue Fruit Smoothie

"This delicious smoothie is sweetened with natural sugars. Replace any of the fruit ingredients with your favorites if you like, but make sure one of them is frozen to make it nice and thick!"
Serving: 5 m | Total Time: 5 m

Ingredients
- 1/2 large banana, cut into pieces and frozen
- 2 large fresh strawberries, rinsed and sliced
- 1/4 cup blueberries
- 1/2 cup milk
- 1 teaspoon vanilla extract
- 2 tablespoons vanilla yogurt
- 2 ice cubes
- Add all ingredients to list

Directions
1. Place the banana pieces, strawberries, blueberries, milk, vanilla extract, yogurt, and ice cubes in a blender. Blend until smooth.

Nutritional Information
- Calories: 192 kcal 10%
- Fat: 3.2 g 5%
- Carbs: 34g 11%
- Protein: 6.8 g 14%
- Cholesterol: 11 mg 4%
- Sodium: 73 mg 3%

Refreshing Banana Drink

Ingredients
- 1 ripe banana
- 3/4 cup almond milk
- 4 ice cubes
- 1 dash ground cinnamon
- 1 dash vanilla extract
- Add all ingredients to list

Directions
1. Blend banana, almond milk, ice cubes, cinnamon, and vanilla extract together in a blender on medium speed until frothy and smooth, about 1 minute.

Nutritional Information
- Calories: 158 kcal 8%
- Fat: 2.4 g 4%

- Carbs: 34.3g 11%
- Protein: 2.1 g 4%
- Cholesterol: 0 mg 0%
- Sodium: 124 mg 5%

Rosy Rhubarb Smoothie

Ingredients
- 1 cup frozen chopped rhubarb
- 1 small banana, cut in chunks
- 1 cup cranberry juice blend
- 1/2 cup vanilla yogurt
- 3 drops red food coloring (optional)
- Add all ingredients to list

Directions
1. Blend rhubarb, banana, cranberry juice blend, vanilla yogurt, and red food coloring in a blender until smooth.

Nutritional Information
- Calories: 192 kcal 10%
- Fat: 1.1 g 2%
- Carbs: 43.7g 14%
- Protein: 4.2 g 8%
- Cholesterol: 3 mg 1%
- Sodium: 46 mg 2%

Secret Ingredient Smoothie

Ingredients
- 3 cups chopped romaine lettuce
- 1/3 cup milk, or more as needed
- 4 frozen strawberries, or more to taste
- 1 frozen banana, cut into chunks
- 1/4 teaspoon vanilla extract, or to taste (optional)
- Add all ingredients to list

Directions

1. Put romaine lettuce into the bottom of a blender pitcher; add enough milk to cover completely and blend on High until smooth.
2. Drop one strawberry at a time into the blender while still running on High and allow the berry to blend completely before adding the next. Blend one banana chunk at a time into the mixture in the same manner as the strawberries. Thin the smoothie with additional milk to keep smoothie blending properly. Blend vanilla extract into the smoothie.

Nutritional Information

- Calories: 200 kcal 10%
- Fat: 2.7 g 4%
- Carbs: 42g 14%
- Protein: 6.5 g 13%
- Cholesterol: 7 mg 2%
- Sodium: 49 mg 2%

Sesame Mango Smoothie

Ingredients

- 1 banana
- 1 cup frozen mango chunks
- 1 small cucumber, roughly chopped
- 2 cups fresh spinach
- 2 tablespoons cashew butter
- 1 teaspoon toasted sesame seeds
- 1 cup water
- Add all ingredients to list

Directions

1. Layer banana, mango, cucumber, spinach, cashew butter, and sesame seeds in a blender, in the order mentioned; add water. Blend until smoothie is desired consistency, adding more water if desired.

Nutritional Information

- Calories: 183 kcal 9%
- Fat: 9.1 g 14%
- Carbs: 24.6g 8%
- Protein: 5.2 g 10%
- Cholesterol: 0 mg 0%
- Sodium: 128 mg 5%

Silky Strawberry Smoothie

Ingredients
- 1 cup fresh strawberries
- 1 banana, sliced
- 1 cup ice
- 1/2 cup silken tofu
- 1 teaspoon agave nectar (optional)
- Add all ingredients to list

Directions
1. Blend strawberries, banana, ice, tofu, and agave nectar together in a blender until smooth.

Nutritional Information
- Calories: 126 kcal 6%
- Fat: 2.1 g 3%
- Carbs: 23.6g 8%
- Protein: 5.4 g 11%
- Cholesterol: 0 mg 0%
- Sodium: 27 mg 1%

Simple Banana Smoothie

Ingredients
- 3/4 cup vanilla yogurt
- 1/2 cup apple juice
- 1 tablespoon honey, or to taste
- 2 ripe bananas
- 1 teaspoon milk, or to taste
- 4 ice cubes
- Add all ingredients to list

Directions
1. Blend yogurt, apple juice, honey, bananas, milk and ice cubes in a blender until smooth.

Nutritional Information
- Calories: 491 kcal 25%
- Fat: 3.3 g 5%
- Carbs: 111.3g 36%
- Protein: 11.9 g 24%
- Cholesterol: 10 mg 3%
- Sodium: 133 mg 5%

Simple Breakfast Smoothie

Ingredients
- 1 cup yogurt
- 1 orange, peeled and broken into sections
- 1 banana, broken into chunks
- 1/4 cup strawberries, or more to taste
- 1/4 cup ice cubes, or as needed
- 1 teaspoon vanilla extract
- 1 teaspoon ground flax seeds (optional)
- Add all ingredients to list

Directions
1. Blend yogurt, orange, banana, strawberries, ice, vanilla extract, and flax seeds together in a blender until smooth.

Nutritional Information
- Calories: 153 kcal 8%
- Fat: 3 g 5%
- Carbs: 24.4g 8%
- Protein: 7.6 g 15%
- Cholesterol: 7 mg 2%
- Sodium: 88 mg 4%

Simple Summer Smoothie

Ingredients
- 1 banana
- 1 cup frozen strawberries
- 1 cup frozen blueberries

- 1 cup frozen cherries
- 4 ice cubes
- 1/2 cup orange juice
- 3/4 cup vanilla yogurt
- 1/2 teaspoon honey (optional)
- Add all ingredients to list

Directions

1. Place the banana, strawberries, blueberries, cherries, and ice cubes into a blender. Pour in the orange juice, vanilla yogurt, and honey. Puree until smooth.

Nutritional Information

- Calories: 139 kcal 7%
- Fat: 1.2 g 2%
- Carbs: 31.1g 10%
- Protein: 3.6 g 7%
- Cholesterol: 2 mg < 1%
- Sodium: 33 mg 1%

Sissy's Frozen Banana and Pumpkin Smoothie

Ingredients

- 3 cups vanilla-flavored almond milk (such as Silk®), or as needed
- 2 bananas, frozen
- 1/2 (15 ounce) can pumpkin puree, frozen into small balls
- 5 tablespoons honey, or to taste
- Add all ingredients to list

Directions

1. Combine almond milk, bananas, pumpkin puree, and honey in a blender. Cover and blend until thick and texture resembles a smoothie, about 3 minutes.

Nutritional Information

- Calories: 397 kcal 20%
- Fat: 4.7 g 7%
- Carbs: 91.6g 30%
- Protein: 4.2 g 8%
- Cholesterol: 0 mg 0%

- Sodium: 500 mg 20%

Skinny Almond Milk Shake

Ingredients
- 15 ice cubes, or as desired
- 3/4 cup almond milk
- 1/3 banana
- 1 tablespoon unsweetened cocoa powder
- 1/2 teaspoon vanilla extract
- Add all ingredients to list

Directions
1. Blend ice cubes, almond milk, banana, cocoa powder, and vanilla extract together in a blender until smooth.

Nutritional Information
- Calories: 102 kcal 5%
- Fat: 2.9 g 4%
- Carbs: 18.6g 6%
- Protein: 2.3 g 5%
- Cholesterol: 0 mg 0%
- Sodium: 131 mg 5%

Smoothie Bowl with Mango and Coconut

Ingredients
- 1 1/2 cups frozen mango chunks
- 1 cup vanilla-flavored almond milk
- 1 frozen banana, chopped
- 1 tablespoon unsweetened coconut cream
- 1/4 teaspoon vanilla extract
- 1 tablespoon flaked coconut
- 1 teaspoon goji berries
- 1/2 teaspoon chia seeds
- Add all ingredients to list

Directions

1. Place mango chunks, almond milk, banana, coconut cream, and vanilla extract in a blender; puree until smoothie is thick and smooth. Pour into a serving bowl.

2. Top smoothie bowl with flaked coconut, goji berries, and chia seeds.

Nutritional Information

- Calories: 442 kcal 22%
- Fat: 10.6 g 16%
- Carbs: 90.3g 29%
- Protein: 4.5 g 9%
- Cholesterol: 0 mg 0%
- Sodium: 181 mg 7%

Smoothie for a Boss!

Ingredients

- 2 cups milk
- 15 slices frozen peach, or more to taste
- 1 banana
- 3 1/2 ounces fruit yogurt
- 2 tablespoons chocolate sauce (optional)
- Add all ingredients to list

Directions

1. Pour milk into a blender; add peaches, banana, and yogurt. Blend mixture until smooth; add chocolate sauce and blend until smooth.

Nutritional Information

- Calories: 294 kcal 15%
- Fat: 5.7 g 9%
- Carbs: 50.6g 16%
- Protein: 11.2 g 22%
- Cholesterol: 21 mg 7%
- Sodium: 145 mg 6%

Spinach and Banana Power Smoothie

Ingredients
- 1 cup plain soy milk
- 3/4 cup packed fresh spinach leaves
- 1 large banana, sliced
- Add all ingredients to list

Directions
1. Blend soy milk and spinach leaves together in a blender until smooth. Add banana and pulse until thoroughly blended.

Nutritional Information
- Calories: 257 kcal 13%
- Fat: 4.8 g 7%
- Carbs: 47.1g 15%
- Protein: 10.1 g 20%
- Cholesterol: 0 mg 0%
- Sodium: 143 mg 6%

Spinach and Berry Smoothie with Truvia® Natural Sweetener

Ingredients
- 1 cup fresh strawberries
- 1 banana
- 1 cup orange juice
- 1 cup almond milk
- 2 cups fresh baby spinach
- 1 cup ice
- 4 (3.5 gram) packets Truvia® natural sweetener, or more to desired level of sweetness
- Add all ingredients to list

Directions
1. Add all ingredients into a blender.
2. Blend on high until smooth.

Nutritional Information
- Calories: 86 kcal 4%
- Fat: 1.1 g 2%
- Carbs: 21.8g 7%
- Protein: 1.7 g 3%
- Cholesterol: 0 mg 0%
- Sodium: 55 mg 2%

Spinach and Kale Smoothie

Ingredients
- 2 cups fresh spinach
- 1 cup almond milk
- 1 tablespoon peanut butter
- 1 tablespoon chia seeds (optional)
- 1 leaf kale
- 1 sliced frozen banana
- Add all ingredients to list

Directions
1. Blend spinach, almond milk, peanut butter, chia seeds, and kale together in a blender until smooth. Add banana and blend until smooth.

Nutritional Information
- Calories: 325 kcal 16%
- Fat: 13.9 g 21%
- Carbs: 46.1g 15%
- Protein: 10 g 20%
- Cholesterol: 0 mg 0%
- Sodium: 293 mg 12%

Strawberry Banana Avocado Smoothie

Ingredients
- 2 tablespoons oats
- 4 ice cubes
- 1 small banana
- 1/2 avocado, peeled and pitted
- 2 strawberries, hulled, or more to taste

- 1 cup carrot juice
- 1 (5.3 ounce) container banana cream yogurt (such as Oikos®)
- Add all ingredients to list

Directions
1. Grind oats in a blender into a powder-like consistency. Add ice cubes; pulse until ground. Add banana, avocado, and strawberries; blend until smooth. Pour in carrot juice and yogurt; blend until combined.

Nutritional Information
- Calories: 336 kcal 17%
- Fat: 3.5 g 5%
- Carbs: 69.7g 22%
- Protein: 10.5 g 21%
- Cholesterol: 3 mg 1%
- Sodium: 160 mg 6%

Strawberry Banana Nutella® Smoothie

Ingredients
- 6 fluid ounces low-fat milk
- 6 ounces plain fat-free Greek yogurt
- 1 banana, sliced
- 4 fresh strawberries
- 2 tablespoons chocolate-hazelnut spread (such as Nutella®)
- Add all ingredients to list

Directions
1. Blend milk, yogurt, banana, strawberries, and chocolate-hazelnut spread together in a blender until smooth.

Nutritional Information
- Calories: 457 kcal 23%
- Fat: 11.4 g 17%
- Carbs: 67.4g 22%
- Protein: 24.9 g 50%
- Cholesterol: 7 mg 2%
- Sodium: 190 mg 8%

Strawberry Banana Peanut Butter Smoothie

"This creamy treat has protein and no added sugar for a yummy breakfast or dessert!"
Serving: *10 m |* **Total Time:** *10 m*

Ingredients
* 1/2 cup nonfat plain yogurt
* 2 tablespoons peanut butter
* 1 banana
* 4 fresh strawberries, hulled
* 10 ice cubes
* Add all ingredients to list

Directions
1. Place yogurt, peanut butter, banana, strawberries, and ice cubes into a blender. Puree until smooth.

Nutritional Information
* Calories: 389 kcal 19%
* Fat: 18.8 g 29%
* Carbs: 45.6g 15%
* Protein: 16.2 g 32%
* Cholesterol: 7 mg 2%
* Sodium: 243 mg 10%

Strawberry Banana Protein Shake

Ingredients
* 1 cup skim milk
* 1 scoop vanilla-flavored whey protein powder
* 2 cups ice
* 1 cup strawberries
* 1 large banana
* 1 tablespoon natural peanut butter
* Add all ingredients to list

Directions

1.   Layer milk, protein powder, ice, strawberries, banana, and peanut butter in a blender in this order; blend until creamy and smooth.

Nutritional Information

*   Calories: 261 kcal 13%
*   Fat: 5.2 g 8%
*   Carbs: 31.1g 10%
*   Protein: 26.1 g 52%
*   Cholesterol: 9 mg 3%
*   Sodium: 187 mg 7%

Strawberry Banana Protein Smoothie

"This balanced smoothie is great for a meal replacement or after a workout."
Serving: *10 m |* **Total Time:** *10 m*

Ingredients

*   1 banana
*   1 1/4 cups sliced fresh strawberries
*   10 whole almonds
*   2 tablespoons water
*   1 cup ice cubes
*   3 tablespoons chocolate flavored protein powder
*   Add all ingredients to list

Directions

1.   Place the banana, strawberries, almonds, and water into a blender. Blend to mix, then add the ice cubes and puree until smooth. Add the protein powder, and continue mixing until evenly incorporated, about 30 seconds.

Nutritional Information

*   Calories: 349 kcal 17%
*   Fat: 8.1 g 12%
*   Carbs: 53.2g 17%
*   Protein: 21 g 42%
*   Cholesterol: 0 mg 0%
*   Sodium: 195 mg 8%

Strawberry Banana Smoothie from Reddi wip®

Ingredients
- 1/2 cup chopped fresh strawberries
- 1/4 medium banana, peeled and halved
- 1/4 cup vanilla nonfat yogurt with low-calorie sweetener
- 1/2 cup crushed ice
- Reddi-wip® Original Dairy Whipped Topping
- Add all ingredients to list

Directions
1. Place strawberries, banana and yogurt in blender container. Pulse until fruit is well blended, scraping sides of container, if necessary.
2. Add ice; pulse until ice is well blended.
3. Pour into glass and top with one serving (2 tablespoons) Reddi-wip. Serve immediately.

Nutritional Information
- Calories: 98 kcal 5%
- Fat: 1.3 g 2%
- Carbs: 19.3g 6%
- Protein: 2.7 g 5%
- Cholesterol: 6 mg 2%
- Sodium: 40 mg 2%

Strawberry Banana Smoothie

"Our whole family starts nearly every day with this thick, delicious smoothie."
Serving: *5 m |* **Total Time:** *5 m*

Ingredients
- 1 1/2 cups vanilla yogurt
- 2 bananas, cut up
- 1/2 cup frozen strawberries
- 2 tablespoons wheat germ
- 1 tablespoon honey
- Add all ingredients to list

Directions

1.   Combine the yogurt, bananas, strawberries, wheat germ, and honey in a blender; blend until smooth, about 1 minute.

Nutritional Information
- Calories: 332 kcal 17%
- Fat: 3.4 g 5%
- Carbs: 68g 22%
- Protein: 12.2 g 24%
- Cholesterol: 9 mg 3%
- Sodium: 124 mg 5%

Strawberry Colada Smoothie

Ingredients
- 1 cup cold coconut water
- 1 cup diced peaches
- 2 kiwis, peeled and sliced
- 1/2 banana
- 5 strawberries
- 1 tablespoon honey
- 1 teaspoon ground ginger
- 1 teaspoon wheat germ
- Add all ingredients to list

Directions

1.   Blend coconut water, peaches, kiwis, banana, strawberries, honey, ground ginger, and wheat germ together in a blender on medium speed until smooth, 30 seconds to 1 minute.

Nutritional Information
- Calories: 328 kcal 16%
- Fat: 2.1 g 3%
- Carbs: 78.6g 25%
- Protein: 5.5 g 11%
- Cholesterol: 0 mg 0%
- Sodium: 265 mg 11%

Strawberry Fields Smoothie

Ingredients
- 2 cups fresh spinach
- 2 cups frozen unsweetened strawberries
- 1 cup chopped cucumber
- 2 carrots, chopped
- 1 banana, cut into chunks
- 1 apple, chopped
- 2/3 cup water
- 1/2 cup ice cubes, or as desired
- 1 tablespoon flax seed, or to taste (optional)
- Add all ingredients to list

Directions
1. Blend spinach, strawberries, cucumber, carrots, banana, apple, water, ice cubes, and flax seed together in a blender until smooth.

Nutritional Information
- Calories: 244 kcal 12%
- Fat: 3.4 g 5%
- Carbs: 55.3g 18%
- Protein: 4.8 g 10%
- Cholesterol: 0 mg 0%
- Sodium: 84 mg 3%

Strawberry Kiwi Smoothie

Ingredients
- 2 cups fresh ripe strawberries, stems removed
- 1 1/2 cups vanilla yogurt
- 1 cup orange juice
- 2 bananas
- 2 kiwis, peeled
- 1/4 cup honey
- Add all ingredients to list

Directions

1. Blend strawberries, yogurt, orange juice, bananas, kiwis, and honey together in a blender until smooth.

Nutritional Information

- Calories: 269 kcal 13%
- Fat: 1.9 g 3%
- Carbs: 61g 20%
- Protein: 6.6 g 13%
- Cholesterol: 5 mg 2%
- Sodium: 65 mg 3%

Strawberry Oatmeal Breakfast Smoothie

"This is a fast vegan smoothie with a deep pink color and a rich, creamy texture. VERY filling, and perfect for people in a rush in the morning. You don't have to give up a good breakfast when it's this fast to make! I use vitamin fortified soy milk."
***Serving:** 5 m | **Total Time:** 5 m*

Ingredients

- 1 cup soy milk
- 1/2 cup rolled oats
- 1 banana, broken into chunks
- 14 frozen strawberries
- 1/2 teaspoon vanilla extract
- 1 1/2 teaspoons white sugar
- Add all ingredients to list

Directions

1. In a blender, combine soy milk, oats, banana and strawberries. Add vanilla and sugar if desired. Blend until smooth. Pour into glasses and serve.

Nutritional Information

- Calories: 236 kcal 12%
- Fat: 3.7 g 6%
- Carbs: 44.9g 14%
- Protein: 7.6 g 15%
- Cholesterol: 0 mg 0%
- Sodium: 65 mg 3%

Strawberry Orange Banana Smoothie

"Orange, banana, and strawberries make up this refreshing smoothie!"
***Serving:** 5 m | **Total Time:** 5 m*

Ingredients
- 3/4 cup orange juice
- 1 cup fresh strawberries
- 1 ripe banana
- ice cubes
- Add all ingredients to list

Directions
1. Blend the orange juice, strawberries, banana, and ice cubes in a blender until smooth and frothy.

Nutritional Information
- Calories: 238 kcal 12%
- Fat: 1.2 g 2%
- Carbs: 58.2g 19%
- Protein: 3.6 g 7%
- Cholesterol: 0 mg 0%
- Sodium: 8 mg < 1%

Strawberry Peach Smoothie from Yoplait®

Ingredients
- 1 cup frozen strawberries
- 1 large banana, peeled and halved
- 1 (5.3 ounce) container Yoplait® Greek 100 Vanilla Yogurt, divided
- 1/4 cup milk
- 1 tablespoon honey (optional)
- 1 cup sliced frozen peaches
- 1/4 cup orange juice
- Add all ingredients to list

Directions

1. Combine the strawberries, half the banana, 1/2 container of yogurt, milk and honey (if using) in a blender and blend until smooth. Pour into 2 glasses and rinse out the blender.
2. Combine the remaining half the banana, remaining yogurt, peaches and orange juice in the blender and blend until smooth. Pour over the strawberry smoothie layer and serve.

Nutritional Information

- Calories: 235 kcal 12%
- Fat: 1 g 2%
- Carbs: 45.9g 15%
- Protein: 9.5 g 19%
- Cholesterol: 2 mg < 1%
- Sodium: 44 mg 2%

Strawberry Yogurt Shake

Ingredients

- 1 (16 ounce) package fresh strawberries, hulled
- 2 bananas, peeled and sliced
- 3 cups ice cubes
- 1 (16 ounce) container plain low-fat yogurt
- Add all ingredients to list

Directions

1. Blend strawberries, bananas, half of the ice cubes, and yogurt in a blender on high until smooth. Add the remaining ice and blend further until smooth again. Serve immediately.

Nutritional Information

- Calories: 321 kcal 16%
- Fat: 4.6 g 7%
- Carbs: 60.4g 19%
- Protein: 14.7 g 29%
- Cholesterol: 14 mg 5%
- Sodium: 173 mg 7%

Summer Sweet Smoothies

Ingredients
- 2 cups cranberry juice
- 2 cups strawberries
- 1 cup blueberries
- 1 cup watermelon chunks
- 1 banana
- 2 fresh figs
- Add all ingredients to list

Directions
1. Process the cranberry juice, strawberries, blueberries, watermelon, banana, and figs in a blender until smooth and creamy. Enjoy immediately or keep cool in refrigerator.

Nutritional Information
- Calories: 168 kcal 8%
- Fat: 0.7 g 1%
- Carbs: 42.3g 14%
- Protein: 1.5 g 3%
- Cholesterol: 0 mg 0%
- Sodium: 5 mg < 1%

Summertime Fruit Smoothie

Ingredients
- 1 cup Greek yogurt
- 1 1/2 cups frozen sliced peaches
- 1 cup frozen raspberries
- 3 1/2 tablespoons raspberry honey
- 3 cups ice
- 1 1/2 cups pineapple chunks
- 1 cup watermelon chunks
- 1 banana
- Add all ingredients to list

Directions

1. Blend yogurt, peaches, raspberries, and honey together in a blender until smooth; add ice, pineapple, watermelon, and banana. Blend until smooth.

Nutritional Information

- Calories: 136 kcal 7%
- Fat: 2.7 g 4%
- Carbs: 28.2g 9%
- Protein: 2.4 g 5%
- Cholesterol: 6 mg 2%
- Sodium: 20 mg < 1%

Sunshine Juice

Ingredients

- 2 oranges, peeled and segmented
- 1/2 cup fresh raspberries
- 1 medium banana, peeled
- 3 fresh mint leaves
- Add all ingredients to list

Directions

1. Juice everything in juice machine. Pour over ice to serve.

Nutritional Information

- Calories: 293 kcal 15%
- Fat: 1.1 g 2%
- Carbs: 73.6g 24%
- Protein: 5 g 10%
- Cholesterol: 0 mg 0%
- Sodium: 1 mg < 1%

Super Fresh Smoothie

Ingredients

- 1 banana
- 4 leaves kale
- 1/2 lime, juiced

- 1 tablespoon honey, or more to taste (optional)
- Add all ingredients to list

Directions

1. Combine banana, kale, lime juice, and honey in a blender; blend until smooth.

Nutritional Information

- Calories: 211 kcal 11%
- Fat: 1 g 1%
- Carbs: 52.9g 17%
- Protein: 4 g 8%
- Cholesterol: 0 mg 0%
- Sodium: 37 mg 1%

Super Green Tea Smoothie

Ingredients

- 1 cup brewed green tea (such as Gold Peak®), chilled
- 1 cup fresh spinach leaves
- 1 kiwi, peeled
- 1/4 avocado
- 1 banana, broken into chunks and frozen
- 1/2 teaspoon grated fresh ginger
- Add all ingredients to list

Directions

1. Combine tea, spinach, kiwi, avocado, banana, and ginger in a blender. Blend until smooth.

Nutritional Information

- Calories: 120 kcal 6%
- Fat: 4.1 g 6%
- Carbs: 22g 7%
- Protein: 2 g 4%
- Cholesterol: 0 mg 0%
- Sodium: 19 mg < 1%

Super Smoothie

Ingredients
- 1 cup frozen blueberries
- 1/2 cup sliced banana
- 1/2 cup sliced peeled cucumber
- 1/2 cup water
- 1/2 cup vanilla yogurt
- 1/2 cup crushed ice, or as needed
- Add all ingredients to list

Directions
1. Blend blueberries, banana, cucumber, water, and yogurt together in a blender until smooth. Add crushed ice and blend until smooth.

Nutritional Information
- Calories: 64 kcal 3%
- Fat: 0.7 g 1%
- Carbs: 13.6g 4%
- Protein: 2 g 4%
- Cholesterol: 2 mg < 1%
- Sodium: 23 mg < 1%

Superfood Chocolate Pudding Smoothie

Ingredients
- 1 small banana, chopped
- 1/2 avocado
- 1/2 cup soy milk
- 2 tablespoons mixed frozen berries
- 2 teaspoons unsweetened cocoa powder
- 2 teaspoons agave nectar
- 1 teaspoon vanilla extract
- Add all ingredients to list

Directions
1. Blend banana, avocado, soy milk, berries, cocoa powder, agave nectar, and vanilla extract together in a blender until smooth.

Nutritional Information
- Calories: 385 kcal 19%
- Fat: 17.8 g 27%
- Carbs: 54.7g 18%
- Protein: 8 g 16%
- Cholesterol: 0 mg 0%
- Sodium: 71 mg 3%

Superfood Green Smoothie

Ingredients
- 1 cup spinach leaves
- 1 cup shredded kale
- 1/2 pear, cut into chunks
- 1/2 large ripe banana, sliced
- 1/2 cup frozen blueberries
- 1/3 cup plain yogurt
- 4 ice cubes
- 2 tablespoons ground flax seeds
- 1/2 cup brewed green tea, chilled, or more to taste
- Add all ingredients to list

Directions
1. Combine spinach, kale, pear, banana, blueberries, yogurt, ice cubes, and ground flax seeds in a blender; pour in tea. Blend on high until mixture is smooth. Mix with a wooden spoon to redistribute ingredients if needed.

Nutritional Information
- Calories: 175 kcal 9%
- Fat: 6.3 g 10%
- Carbs: 27.4g 9%
- Protein: 5.9 g 12%
- Cholesterol: 2 mg < 1%
- Sodium: 54 mg 2%

Supergirl Summer Smoothie

Ingredients

- 2 bananas, broken into chunks
- 1 cup cubed papaya (optional)
- 1 cup cubed fresh pineapple
- 1 cup cubed honeydew
- 1 cup seedless grapes (optional)
- 3 cubes ice cubes (optional)
- 2 (6 ounce) containers fruit flavored yogurt
- 1/2 cup orange juice, or as needed
- Add all ingredients to list

Directions

1. Place bananas, papaya, pineapple, honeydew, grapes, ice cubes, and yogurt into the bowl of a blender. Pour in orange juice. Cover and puree until smooth, adding additional orange juice if needed to achieve desired consistency.

Nutritional Information

- Calories: 148 kcal 7%
- Fat: 0.5 g < 1%
- Carbs: 34.4g 11%
- Protein: 4.1 g 8%
- Cholesterol: < 1 mg < 1%
- Sodium: 47 mg 2%

Sweet Potato and Banana Smoothie

Ingredients

- 1 large sweet potato
- 1 banana
- 2 cups soy milk
- 1/4 teaspoon ground cinnamon
- Add all ingredients to list

Directions

1. Preheat oven to 350 degrees F (175 degrees C).

2. Bake sweet potato in the preheated oven until tender and cooked through, about 1 hour. Remove peel from cooked sweet potato and cool in the refrigerator 8 hours or overnight.
3. Blend sweet potato, banana, soy milk, and cinnamon together in a blender until smooth.

Nutritional Information
- Calories: 380 kcal 19%
- Fat: 4.6 g 7%
- Carbs: 74.6g 24%
- Protein: 12.2 g 24%
- Cholesterol: 0 mg 0%
- Sodium: 249 mg 10%

Sweet Potato Banana Smoothie

Ingredients
- 1 small banana
- 1/2 small cooked sweet potato
- 1/2 cup cottage cheese
- 1/2 cup low-fat milk
- 5 cubes ice, or as needed
- 1 tablespoon cocoa powder
- 1 tablespoon molasses
- 1 tablespoon honey
- 1/8 teaspoon almond extract
- Add all ingredients to list

Directions
1. Blend banana, sweet potato, cottage cheese, milk, ice, cocoa powder, molasses, honey, and almond extract together in a high-power blender (such as Ninja(R)) until smooth.

Nutritional Information
- Calories: 455 kcal 23%
- Fat: 8.7 g 13%
- Carbs: 78.8g 25%
- Protein: 21.4 g 43%
- Cholesterol: 27 mg 9%
- Sodium: 659 mg 26%

Tasty Breakfast Smoothie

Ingredients
- 1 cup milk
- 1 banana, cut into chunks
- 2 fresh apricots, peeled and pitted
- 1/2 cup plain yogurt
- 2 teaspoons wheat germ
- 2 teaspoons oat bran
- 2 teaspoons maple syrup, or more to taste
- Add all ingredients to list

Directions
1. Blend milk, banana, apricots, yogurt, wheat germ, oat bran, and maple syrup in a blender until smooth and frothy.

Nutritional Information
- Calories: 200 kcal 10%
- Fat: 4.1 g 6%
- Carbs: 34.4g 11%
- Protein: 9.3 g 19%
- Cholesterol: 13 mg 4%
- Sodium: 95 mg 4%

The Best Post Workout Shake

Ingredients
- 1 scoop whey protein powder
- 1 tablespoon flax seed meal
- 1 tablespoon unsweetened cocoa powder
- 1 teaspoon brown sugar (optional)
- 1 cup unsweetened almond milk
- 1 banana
- 1/2 cup frozen mixed berries
- 1 tablespoon smooth peanut butter
- Add all ingredients to list

Directions

1. Layer protein powder, flax meal, cocoa powder, and brown sugar in a blender; add almond milk, banana, berries, and peanut butter. Blend until smooth, about 1 minute.

Nutritional Information

- Calories: 493 kcal 25%
- Fat: 16.5 g 25%
- Carbs: 66.8g 22%
- Protein: 29.2 g 58%
- Cholesterol: 0 mg 0%
- Sodium: 208 mg 8%

The Most Awesome Smoothie You'll Ever Make

Ingredients

- 1 banana
- 1/2 apple
- 1 kiwi, peeled
- 1/2 cup frozen mixed berries
- 1 cup orange juice
- 1/2 cup soy milk
- 1/2 cup nonfat plain yogurt
- 1/2 cup tofu
- 3 tablespoons unsalted natural peanut butter
- 2 tablespoons aloe vera juice
- 2 tablespoons flaxseed oil
- 1 teaspoon barley grass powder (optional)
- Add all ingredients to list

Directions

1. In a blender, combine banana, apple, kiwi, mixed berries and orange juice. Blend until smooth. Add soy milk, yogurt, tofu, peanut butter, aloe vera juice, flaxseed oil, and barley grass powder. Blend again until well blended. Pour into glasses and serve.

Nutritional Information

- Calories: 197 kcal 10%
- Fat: 10.2 g 16%
- Carbs: 22.6g 7%

- Protein: 6.5 g 13%
- Cholesterol: < 1 mg < 1%
- Sodium: 30 mg 1%

Thick and Creamy Banana Yogurt Smoothie

Ingredients
- 1 cup plain yogurt, or more to taste
- 1 banana, sliced and frozen
- 3 tablespoons honey
- 2 tablespoons orange juice
- 1 tablespoon almond butter
- Add all ingredients to list

Directions
1. Blend yogurt, bananas, honey, orange juice, and almond butter in a blender until smooth.

Nutritional Information
- Calories: 283 kcal 14%
- Fat: 6.9 g 11%
- Carbs: 51.4g 17%
- Protein: 8.5 g 17%
- Cholesterol: 7 mg 2%
- Sodium: 124 mg 5%

Thin Mint Green Monster

Ingredients
- 1/2 cup chilled coconut milk
- 1 cup fresh spinach leaves
- 10 leaves fresh mint, chopped
- 1/4 cup raw cacao seeds
- 1 teaspoon peppermint extract
- 1 (1 gram) packet stevia powder
- 1 banana, cut into pieces and frozen
- ice, or as needed
- water, or as needed

- Add all ingredients to list

Directions

1. Blend coconut milk, spinach, mint leaves, cacao seeds, peppermint extract, and stevia powder in a blender. While blender is running, drop in banana chunks, one by one. Add ice cubes until smoothie has desired thickness, and water if smoothie is too thick.

Nutritional Information

- Calories: 173 kcal 9%
- Fat: 12.3 g 19%
- Carbs: 16.2g 5%
- Protein: 2.2 g 4%
- Cholesterol: 0 mg 0%
- Sodium: 21 mg < 1%

Tofuberry Smoothie

Ingredients

- 1/4 cup diced silken tofu
- 2 tablespoons soy milk
- 1/4 cup fruit yogurt
- 1/2 cup raspberries
- 1/4 banana
- 2 cups orange juice
- Add all ingredients to list

Directions

1. Place tofu, soy milk, yogurt, raspberries, banana, and orange juice in a blender. Blend until smooth. Pour in glasses over ice or vanilla ice cream.

Nutritional Information

- Calories: 132 kcal 7%
- Fat: 1.4 g 2%
- Carbs: 26.8g 9%
- Protein: 4.1 g 8%
- Cholesterol: < 1 mg < 1%
- Sodium: 26 mg 1%

Triple Threat Fruit Smoothie

"A wonderful, delightful fruit smoothie...it will help you cool down after a hot day in the sun."
Serving: *5 m* | **Total Time:** *5 m*

Ingredients
- 1 kiwi, sliced
- 1 banana, peeled and chopped
- 1/2 cup blueberries
- 1 cup strawberries
- 1 cup ice cubes
- 1/2 cup orange juice
- 1 (8 ounce) container peach yogurt
- Add all ingredients to list

Directions
1. In a blender, blend the kiwi, banana, blueberries, strawberries, ice, orange juice, and yogurt until smooth.

Nutritional Information
- Calories: 134 kcal 7%
- Fat: 1.1 g 2%
- Carbs: 29.6g 10%
- Protein: 3.6 g 7%
- Cholesterol: 4 mg 1%
- Sodium: 41 mg 2%

Tropical Cooler Smoothie

Ingredients
- 1 cup orange juice
- 2 cups pineapple chunks, drained
- 1 banana, coarsely chopped
- 1/4 cup skim milk
- 2 tablespoons honey
- 1 cup crushed ice
- Add all ingredients to list

Directions

1. In a blender combine orange juice, pineapple chunks, milk, honey and crushed ice. Blend until smooth.

Nutritional Information

- Calories: 339 kcal 17%
- Fat: 0.7 g 1%
- Carbs: 86g 28%
- Protein: 3.7 g 7%
- Cholesterol: < 1 mg < 1%
- Sodium: 20 mg < 1%

Tropical Smoothie with Kale

Ingredients

- 1 1/2 cups frozen pineapple chunks
- 1 cup chopped kale
- 1 banana, cut in chunks
- 1 cup almond milk, or as needed
- Add all ingredients to list

Directions

1. Place pineapple, kale, and banana in a NutriBullet(R) or blender; add almond milk. Blend until smooth.

Nutritional Information

- Calories: 163 kcal 8%
- Fat: 1.9 g 3%
- Carbs: 37.3g 12%
- Protein: 2.9 g 6%
- Cholesterol: 0 mg 0%
- Sodium: 96 mg 4%

Tropical Sunshine Smoothie

Ingredients

- 1 banana
- 1/2 cup orange juice

- 1/2 cup cubed fresh mango
- 1/2 cup cubed fresh pineapple
- 1/2 cup coconut water
- 1/2 teaspoon freshly squeezed lime juice
- 1 sprig fresh chocolate mint, finely chopped
- Add all ingredients to list

Directions
1. Blend banana, orange juice, mango, pineapple, coconut water, lime juice, mint in a blender until smooth.

Nutritional Information
- Calories: 140 kcal 7%
- Fat: 0.6 g < 1%
- Carbs: 34.8g 11%
- Protein: 2 g 4%
- Cholesterol: 0 mg 0%
- Sodium: 66 mg 3%

Turmeric Mango Smoothie

Ingredients
- 2 banana, broken into chunks
- 1 cup frozen mango chunks
- 2 tablespoons cashew butter
- 1/8 teaspoon ground turmeric
- 2 cups water
- Add all ingredients to list

Directions
1. Combine bananas, mango, cashew butter, and turmeric powder in a blender; add water. Blend mixture until smooth.

Nutritional Information
- Calories: 253 kcal 13%
- Fat: 8.5 g 13%
- Carbs: 45.5g 15%
- Protein: 4.5 g 9%
- Cholesterol: 0 mg 0%

- Sodium: 12 mg < 1%

Twisted Colada Protein Smoothie

Ingredients
- 1/2 cup shredded coconut
- 8 almonds
- 2 tablespoons flax seeds
- 1 tablespoon chia seeds
- 1 cup sliced frozen banana
- 1 cup coconut milk beverage (such as Silk®)
- 2 fresh pineapple spears
- 2 tablespoons protein powder
- 1 teaspoon agave nectar
- Add all ingredients to list

Directions
1. Blend coconut, almonds, flax seeds, and chia seeds together in a blender or food processor until slightly smooth. Add banana, coconut milk beverage, pineapple, protein powder, and agave nectar; blend until smooth.

Nutritional Information
- Calories: 462 kcal 23%
- Fat: 19 g 29%
- Carbs: 67g 22%
- Protein: 14.1 g 28%
- Cholesterol: 0 mg 0%
- Sodium: 64 mg 3%

Uncle Monkey Smoothie

Ingredients
- 2 bananas, cut into small chunks
- 1/4 cup vanilla yogurt
- 5 ice cubes
- 3 tablespoons peanut butter
- 2 tablespoons milk
- 1 tablespoon white sugar

- Add all ingredients to list

Directions
1. Blend bananas, yogurt, ice cubes, peanut butter, milk, and sugar together in a blender until smooth.

Nutritional Information
- Calories: 153 kcal 8%
- Fat: 6.7 g 10%
- Carbs: 21.5g 7%
- Protein: 4.7 g 9%
- Cholesterol: 1 mg < 1%
- Sodium: 71 mg 3%

Vanilla Banamango Smoothie

Ingredients
- 1/4 cup orange juice, or to taste
- 1 mango, sliced
- 1 frozen banana, sliced
- 2 baby carrots
- 1 (6 ounce) container vanilla yogurt
- 2 ice cubes, or as desired
- 1 teaspoon ground ginger
- Add all ingredients to list

Directions
1. Pour orange juice into the pitcher of a blender and add mango, frozen banana, carrots, vanilla yogurt, ice cubes, and ginger. Pulse several times to crush ice, then blend until smooth, 30 seconds to 1 minute.

Nutritional Information
- Calories: 192 kcal 10%
- Fat: 1.6 g 2%
- Carbs: 42.1g 14%
- Protein: 5.5 g 11%
- Cholesterol: 4 mg 1%
- Sodium: 62 mg 2%

Vanilla Banana Smoothie

Ingredients
- 2 bananas, broken into chunks
- 1 cup vanilla ice cream
- 1/2 teaspoon vanilla extract
- 1/2 cup fresh orange juice
- 1 cup milk
- Add all ingredients to list

Directions
1. Place banana and vanilla ice cream into a blender. Pour in vanilla extract, orange juice, and milk. Puree until thick and smooth.

Nutritional Information
- Calories: 165 kcal 8%
- Fat: 5.1 g 8%
- Carbs: 27.4g 9%
- Protein: 4 g 8%
- Cholesterol: 19 mg 6%
- Sodium: 52 mg 2%

Vegan Chocolate Hemp High Fiber Smoothie

Ingredients
- 8 fluid ounces coconut water
- 1 sliced frozen banana
- 1/2 cup ice cubes, or as desired
- 3 tablespoons hemp protein powder
- 1 tablespoon cocoa powder
- Add all ingredients to list

Directions
1. Blend coconut water, banana, ice, hemp protein powder, and cocoa powder together in a blender until smooth.

Nutritional Information
- Calories: 281 kcal 14%

- Fat: 5.1 g 8%
- Carbs: 45.5g 15%
- Protein: 19 g 38%
- Cholesterol: 0 mg 0%
- Sodium: 265 mg 11%

Vegan Green Smoothie

Ingredients
- 2 cups coconut water
- 1 cup baby spinach
- 1 banana
- 6 sliced fresh strawberries
- 5 dates, pitted
- Add all ingredients to list

Directions
1. Blend coconut water, spinach, banana, strawberries, and dates together in a blender.

Nutritional Information
- Calories: 118 kcal 6%
- Fat: 0.7 g 1%
- Carbs: 28.4g 9%
- Protein: 2.4 g 5%
- Cholesterol: 0 mg 0%
- Sodium: 177 mg 7%

Vegan Morning Smoothie

Ingredients
- 1 banana
- 1/3 cup frozen chopped spinach
- 1/2 cup frozen mixed fruit
- 1 tablespoon flax seed meal
- 1/2 scoop vegan protein powder
- 1 tablespoon chia seeds
- 1/2 teaspoon matcha green tea powder

- water to cover
- Add all ingredients to list

Directions

1. Layer banana, spinach, mixed fruit, flax meal, protein powder, chia seeds, and matcha powder in a blender in the order listed; add enough water to cover. Cover blender and blend until smooth.

Nutritional Information

- Calories: 352 kcal 18%
- Fat: 6.7 g 10%
- Carbs: 53.5g 17%
- Protein: 25.5 g 51%
- Cholesterol: 6 mg 2%
- Sodium: 164 mg 7%

Vegan Strawberry Oatmeal Breakfast Smoothie

Ingredients

- 1 cup almond milk
- 1/2 cup rolled oats
- 14 frozen strawberries
- 1 banana, broken into chunks
- 1 1/2 teaspoons agave nectar (optional)
- 1/2 teaspoon vanilla extract (optional)
- Add all ingredients to list

Directions

1. Blend almond milk, oats, strawberries, banana, agave nectar, and vanilla extract in a blender until smooth.

Nutritional Information

- Calories: 205 kcal 10%
- Fat: 2.9 g 5%
- Carbs: 42.4g 14%
- Protein: 4.2 g 8%
- Cholesterol: 0 mg 0%
- Sodium: 83 mg 3%

Veggie Fruit and Nut Nutritious Green Smoothie!

Ingredients
- 1 1/2 cups baby spinach leaves
- 1 cup shredded carrots
- 1/2 cup sliced raw beet
- 1/2 pear, cored and chopped
- 1/2 cup milk
- 1/2 banana, sliced
- 1/4 cup cottage cheese
- 1/4 cup walnut halves
- 1/4 cup whole almonds
- 2 tablespoons Greek yogurt
- 1 tablespoon honey
- 1/2 teaspoon ground cinnamon
- Add all ingredients to list

Directions
1. Blend spinach, carrots, beet, pear, milk, banana, cottage cheese, walnuts, almonds, yogurt, honey, and cinnamon together in a blender until smooth.

Nutritional Information
- Calories: 386 kcal 19%
- Fat: 21.3 g 33%
- Carbs: 40.9g 13%
- Protein: 14.2 g 28%
- Cholesterol: 12 mg 4%
- Sodium: 231 mg 9%

Very Berry Blueberry Smoothie

Ingredients
- 1 banana, chopped
- 1 kiwi, sliced
- 3/4 cup blueberries
- 1 cup ice cubes
- 1 (8 ounce) container vanilla yogurt
- Add all ingredients to list

Directions

1. Combine the banana, kiwi, blueberries, ice cubes, and vanilla yogurt in a blender; blend until smooth.

Nutritional Information

- Calories: 135 kcal 7%
- Fat: 1.3 g 2%
- Carbs: 28.4g 9%
- Protein: 4.7 g 9%
- Cholesterol: 4 mg 1%
- Sodium: 54 mg 2%

Very Berry Tea Smoothie

Ingredients

- 1 cup brewed black tea (such as Gold Peak®), chilled
- 1 cup frozen mixed berries
- 1 cup frozen pineapple chunks
- 1 banana, broken into chunks and frozen
- 1/2 lemon, juiced
- 3 fresh mint leaves, or more to taste
- 1 teaspoon honey (optional)
- Add all ingredients to list

Directions

1. Combine tea, berries, pineapple, banana, lemon juice, mint, and honey in a blender. Blend until smooth.

Nutritional Information

- Calories: 298 kcal 15%
- Fat: 0.6 g < 1%
- Carbs: 77.3g 25%
- Protein: 3.2 g 6%
- Cholesterol: 0 mg 0%
- Sodium: 11 mg < 1%

Very Orange Smoothie without Oranges

Ingredients
- 1 mango - peeled, seeded, and chopped
- 2 carrots, cut into chunks
- 1 banana, chopped
- 1 yellow bell pepper, chopped, or to taste
- 1/2 red bell pepper, chopped, or more to taste
- 1 ounce chilled mineral water, or as needed
- 1 teaspoon lemon juice, or to taste
- 1 teaspoon honey, or to taste (optional)
- 1 teaspoon chia seeds, or to taste (optional)
- Add all ingredients to list

Directions
1. Blend mango, carrots, banana, yellow bell pepper, red bell pepper, mineral water, lemon juice, honey, or chia seeds in a blender until smooth. Add more water for a thinner consistency.

Nutritional Information
- Calories: 87 kcal 4%
- Fat: 0.6 g < 1%
- Carbs: 21.3g 7%
- Protein: 1.4 g 3%
- Cholesterol: 0 mg 0%
- Sodium: 28 mg 1%

Yam Smoothie

Ingredients
- 2 medium yams
- 3 cups vanilla yogurt
- 1 cup milk
- 2 cups ice cubes
- 1 teaspoon white sugar
- 1 ripe banana, sliced
- Add all ingredients to list

Directions

1. Prick yams with a fork, and place on a plate. Cook in the microwave for 8 to 10 minutes, turning once, until tender. Cool, peel and dice.
2. Combine the yams, yogurt, milk, ice cubes, sugar and banana in the container of a blender. Blend until smooth.

Nutritional Information
- Calories: 226 kcal 11%
- Fat: 2 g 3%
- Carbs: 45.9g 15%
- Protein: 7.2 g 14%
- Cholesterol: 7 mg 2%
- Sodium: 84 mg 3%

Yummy Mango Banana Milkshake

Ingredients
- 1/2 small mango - peeled, seeded and diced
- 1 banana, cut in chunks
- 1 scoop vanilla ice cream (optional)
- 1 tablespoon white sugar, or to taste
- 1/8 teaspoon ground cinnamon, or to taste
- 1 pinch ground nutmeg, or to taste
- 2 cups milk
- Add all ingredients to list

Directions

1. Place mango, banana, and ice cream into a blender, and sprinkle with white sugar, cinnamon, and nutmeg. Pour in milk and place the lid on the blender. Blend until smooth, then pour into cups to serve.

Nutritional Information
- Calories: 124 kcal 6%
- Fat: 3.2 g 5%
- Carbs: 20.2g 7%
- Protein: 4.6 g 9%
- Cholesterol: 12 mg 4%
- Sodium: 55 mg 2%

Chapter 4: Blueberry Smoothies

***

All Fruit Smoothies

"Quick, easy smoothies made entirely with fruit!"
***Serving:** 10 m | **Total Time:** 10 m*

Ingredients
- 1 cup pineapple juice
- 1 large banana, cut into chunks
- 1 cup frozen strawberries
- 1 cup frozen blueberries
- Add all ingredients to list

Directions
1. Pour pineapple juice into a blender and add banana, strawberries, and blueberries. Cover and blend until smooth, about 1 minute. Pour into 2 glasses.

Nutritional Information
- Calories: 205 kcal 10%
- Fat: 1 g 2%
- Carbs: 51.1g 16%
- Protein: 2 g 4%
- Cholesterol: 0 mg 0%
- Sodium: 6 mg < 1%

Almond Berry Smoothie

"Almond milk and almond butter are the star ingredients in this berry smoothie for a nutritious, on-the-go meal that is vegan and paleo-friendly."
***Serving:** 10 m | **Total Time:** 10 m*

Ingredients
- 1 cup frozen blueberries
- 1 banana
- 1/2 cup almond milk
- 1 tablespoon almond butter
- water as needed

- Add all ingredients to list

Directions

1. Combine blueberries, banana, almond milk, and almond butter in a blender; blend until smooth, adding water for a thinner smoothie.

Nutritional Information

- Calories: 321 kcal 16%
- Fat: 11.7 g 18%
- Carbs: 55.6g 18%
- Protein: 5.3 g 11%
- Cholesterol: 0 mg 0%
- Sodium: 162 mg 6%

Almond Butter and Blueberry Smoothie

"My almond butter and jelly smoothie is a spin-off of 'peanut butter and jelly' and it is my perfect mid-afternoon snack or sometimes even my lunch!"
Serving: *10 m |* **Total Time:** *10 m*

Ingredients

- 1 cup almond milk
- 1 cup blueberries
- 4 ice cubes, or more to taste
- 1 scoop vanilla protein powder
- 1 tablespoon almond butter, or more to taste
- 1 tablespoon chia seeds, or more to taste
- Add all ingredients to list

Directions

1. Blend almond milk, blueberries, ice cubes, vanilla protein powder, almond butter, and chia seeds in a blender until smooth.

Nutritional Information

- Calories: 230 kcal 11%
- Fat: 8.1 g 12%
- Carbs: 20g 6%
- Protein: 21.6 g 43%
- Cholesterol: 6 mg 2%

- Sodium: 225 mg 9%

Amy's Healthy Fruity

"This is the type of smoothie that you can throw together quickly for a meal or snack."
***Serving:** 10 m | **Total Time:** 10 m*

Ingredients
- 1 cup strawberries, hulled
- 1/3 cup frozen blueberries
- 2 bananas, peeled and cut into chunks
- 1/2 cup orange juice
- 1 1/2 cups plain yogurt
- 1 tablespoon soy milk powder
- Add all ingredients to list

Directions
1. Combine strawberries, blueberries, bananas, orange juice, yogurt, and soy milk powder in a blender. Blend until smooth, then pour into glasses and serve.

Nutritional Information
- Calories: 155 kcal 8%
- Fat: 2.2 g 3%
- Carbs: 29.5g 10%
- Protein: 6.2 g 12%
- Cholesterol: 6 mg 2%
- Sodium: 78 mg 3%

Ann's Berry Green Smoothie

Ingredients
- 2 cups frozen strawberries
- 1 1/2 cups warm water
- 2 cups milk
- 1 1/2 cups fresh spinach, or to taste
- 1 cup frozen blueberries
- 1 frozen chopped banana
- 1 tablespoon honey

- 1/2 lemon, juiced
- Add all ingredients to list

Directions
1. Place strawberries in a bowl; add warm water.
2. Blend milk and spinach together in a blender until smooth. Add blueberries, banana, and honey and blend until smooth. Add strawberries-water mixture and lemon juice and blend until smooth.

Nutritional Information
- Calories: 303 kcal 15%
- Fat: 5.7 g 9%
- Carbs: 57.4g 19%
- Protein: 10.3 g 21%
- Cholesterol: 20 mg 7%
- Sodium: 128 mg 5%

Avocado Blueberry Banana and Chia Smoothie

Ingredients
- 1 cup vanilla-flavored almond milk
- 1 avocado - peeled, pitted, and halved
- 1 cup fresh blueberries
- 1 banana
- 1 cup ice
- 1 tablespoon chia seeds
- Add all ingredients to list

Directions
1. Combine almond milk, avocado, blueberries, banana, ice, and chia seeds in a blender; blend until smooth.

Nutritional Information
- Calories: 643 kcal 32%
- Fat: 35.3 g 54%
- Carbs: 85.6g 28%
- Protein: 8.6 g 17%
- Cholesterol: 0 mg 0%
- Sodium: 182 mg 7%

Avocado Blueberry Smoothie

"It's not GREEN, so my kids love it! No sweetener needed; the blueberries do the trick. Very delicious and nutritious! If you use fresh blueberries, you may want to add ice but frozen blueberries makes it the perfect consistency."
***Serving:** 5 m | **Total Time:** 5 m*

Ingredients
- 1 cup frozen blueberries
- 1 (6 ounce) container plain Greek-style yogurt
- 1/2 cup almond milk
- 1/2 cup water
- 1/4 avocado - peeled, pitted, and diced
- Add all ingredients to list

Directions
1. Blend blueberries, yogurt, almond milk, water, and avocado in a blender until smooth.

Nutritional Information
- Calories: 297 kcal 15%
- Fat: 12.3 g 19%
- Carbs: 39.2g 13%
- Protein: 11 g 22%
- Cholesterol: 10 mg 3%
- Sodium: 206 mg 8%

Backyard Berry Bowl

Ingredients
- 1 cup ice cubes, or as needed
- 1 cup strawberries, divided
- 2 bananas, sliced, divided
- 1/2 cup blackberries
- 1/4 cup apple juice
- 1/2 cup blueberries
- 1/2 cup granola
- 1 teaspoon honey, or to taste

- Add all ingredients to list

Directions
1. Blend ice, 1/2 cup strawberries, 1 banana, blackberries, and apple juice together in a blender until smooth, adding more ice depending on your desired consistency. Pour smoothie into a bowl.
2. Top smoothie with remaining strawberries, remaining banana, blueberries, and granola. Drizzle honey over the top.

Nutritional Information
- Calories: 341 kcal 17%
- Fat: 8.3 g 13%
- Carbs: 64.5g 21%
- Protein: 7.1 g 14%
- Cholesterol: 0 mg 0%
- Sodium: 15 mg < 1%

Banana Berry Smoothie with Truvia® Natural Sweetener

Ingredients
- 1 cup strawberries
- 1 cup blueberries
- 1 banana
- 1 cup fat-free plain yogurt
- 1 cup orange juice
- 1 cup ice
- 1 tablespoon Truvia® natural sweetener spoonable, plus
- 1/2 teaspoon Truvia® natural sweetener spoonable*
- Add all ingredients to list

Directions
1. Add all ingredients to blender. Blend on high until smooth.
2. Enjoy.

Nutritional Information
- Calories: 121 kcal 6%
- Fat: 0.6 g < 1%
- Carbs: 29.7g 10%
- Protein: 4.8 g 10%

- Cholesterol: 1 mg < 1%
- Sodium: 51 mg 2%

Banana Blueberry Peanut Butter Smoothie

Ingredients
- 1 cup nonfat milk
- 1 cup fresh blueberries
- 5 ice cubes
- 1 banana
- 1 tablespoon vanilla yogurt, or more to taste
- 1 tablespoon natural peanut butter
- 1 scoop chocolate-flavored whey protein powder
- Add all ingredients to list

Directions
1. Combine milk, blueberries, ice cubes, banana, vanilla yogurt, peanut butter, and chocolate protein powder in a blender; blend until smooth.

Nutritional Information
- Calories: 226 kcal 11%
- Fat: 5.1 g 8%
- Carbs: 34.6g 11%
- Protein: 14.1 g 28%
- Cholesterol: 23 mg 8%
- Sodium: 122 mg 5%

Beet and Berry Smoothie

Ingredients
- 1 cup fresh spinach
- 1 beet, peeled and cut into quarters
- 1/2 cup plain Greek yogurt
- 1/2 cup frozen unsweetened red raspberries
- 1/2 cup frozen blueberries
- 1/2 cup ice cubes
- 4 slices cucumber

- Add all ingredients to list

Directions

1. Blend spinach, beet, yogurt, raspberries, blueberries, ice cubes, and cucumber together in a blender until smooth.

Nutritional Information

- Calories: 256 kcal 13%
- Fat: 10.9 g 17%
- Carbs: 33.5g 11%
- Protein: 9.8 g 20%
- Cholesterol: 22 mg 8%
- Sodium: 159 mg 6%

Berry Chocolate Candy Bar Smoothie

Ingredients

- 2 cups chopped kale
- 1 1/2 cups frozen blueberries
- 1 1/2 cups whole milk
- 1 1/2 cups apple juice
- 1 cup frozen raspberries
- 1/4 cup maple syrup, or more to taste
- 2 tablespoons unsweetened cocoa powder, or more to taste
- 1 teaspoon vanilla extract
- 2 pinches sea salt
- Add all ingredients to list

Directions

1. Blend kale, blueberries, milk, apple juice, raspberries, maple syrup, cocoa powder, vanilla extract, and sea salt together in a blender until smooth.

Nutritional Information

- Calories: 270 kcal 14%
- Fat: 4.2 g 6%
- Carbs: 56.6g 18%
- Protein: 5.3 g 11%
- Cholesterol: 9 mg 3%
- Sodium: 217 mg 9%

Berry Coconut Smoothie

Ingredients
- 1 banana
- 1/2 cup frozen blueberries
- 1 tablespoon almond butter
- 1 tablespoon unsweetened flaked coconut
- 1/2 cup water, or as needed
- Add all ingredients to list

Directions
1. Layer banana, blueberries, almond butter, coconut, and water in a blender; blend until smooth, adding more water for a thinner smoothie.

Nutritional Information
- Calories: 286 kcal 14%
- Fat: 13.9 g 21%
- Carbs: 42.2g 14%
- Protein: 4.6 g 9%
- Cholesterol: 0 mg 0%
- Sodium: 80 mg 3%

Berry Good Smoothie II

"A delicious way to get your '5-a-day.' It's a quick and easy breakfast, but great any time of day! Nectarines, strawberries, and blueberries blended with nonfat milk and ice!"
Serving: 10 m | Total Time: 10 m

Ingredients
- 1 nectarine, pitted
- 3/4 cup strawberries, hulled
- 3/4 cup blueberries, rinsed and drained
- 1/3 cup nonfat dry milk powder
- 1 cup crushed ice
- Add all ingredients to list

Directions

1. In a blender combine nectarine, strawberries, blueberries, milk powder and crushed ice. Blend until smooth. pour into glasses and serve.

Nutritional Information

- Calories: 151 kcal 8%
- Fat: 0.7 g 1%
- Carbs: 29.6g 10%
- Protein: 8.7 g 17%
- Cholesterol: 4 mg 1%
- Sodium: 110 mg 4%

Berry Good Smoothie

"This is a naturally sweetened fruit drink. It is great for hot summer days."
Serving: 5 m | **Total Time:** 5 m

Ingredients

- 16 cubes ice
- 1/2 cup water
- 1/2 cup mixed berry fruit juice
- 1/2 cup frozen red raspberries
- 2 1/4 cups frozen mixed berries
- 1/4 cup frozen blueberries
- Add all ingredients to list

Directions

1. Blend 16 ice cubes in a blender until crushed. Pour in water and juice. Blend. Pour in frozen berries. Blend until smooth. Pour into chilled glasses.

Nutritional Information

- Calories: 118 kcal 6%
- Fat: 0.6 g < 1%
- Carbs: 28.9g 9%
- Protein: 1.8 g 4%
- Cholesterol: 0 mg 0%
- Sodium: 9 mg < 1%

Berry nana Soy Smoothie

Ingredients
- 1 cup vanilla soymilk
- 1 cup frozen blueberries or frozen berry mix
- 1 banana, sliced
- 1 tablespoon soy protein powder
- 1/2 cup ice cubes
- 1 teaspoon honey (optional)
- Add all ingredients to list

Directions
1. Puree all ingredients in blender on high until smooth. Serve immediately.

Nutritional Information
- Calories: 172 kcal 9%
- Fat: 2.3 g 4%
- Carbs: 33.1g 11%
- Protein: 7.2 g 14%
- Cholesterol: 0 mg 0%
- Sodium: 88 mg 4%

Berry Smoothie Bowl

Ingredients
- Smoothie:
- 1 cup frozen strawberries
- 1 cup frozen pineapple chunks
- 1 cup plain Greek yogurt
- 1/2 cup coconut water
- 2 tablespoons frozen acai berry pulp, or as desired
- Toppings:
- 1 kiwi, peeled and sliced
- 1/2 banana, sliced
- 1/2 cup fresh blueberries
- 1/2 cup fresh raspberries
- 2 tablespoons sliced almonds
- 2 tablespoons granola
- 1 teaspoon chia seeds (optional)

- Add all ingredients to list

Directions

1. Blend strawberries, pineapple, yogurt, coconut water, and acai pulp in a blender until smooth; pour into a bowl. Top smoothie with kiwi, banana, blueberries, raspberries, almonds, granola, and chia seeds.

Nutritional Information

- Calories: 394 kcal 20%
- Fat: 16.8 g 26%
- Carbs: 54.4g 18%
- Protein: 11.2 g 22%
- Cholesterol: 22 mg 8%
- Sodium: 138 mg 6%

Black and Blueberry Smoothie

"I created this smoothie to keep me going in the morning and prepare for heavy workouts. It's high in good fat and antioxidants and will actually fill you up through the morning. It is also dairy-free."
Serving: *10 m |* **Total Time:** *10 m*

Ingredients

- 1 cup unsweetened almond milk
- 1/2 cup frozen blackberries
- 1/2 cup frozen blueberries
- 2 tablespoons coconut butter
- 1 tablespoon honey
- 1 tablespoon chia seeds
- Add all ingredients to list

Directions

1. Blend almond milk, blackberries, blueberries, coconut butter, honey, and chia seeds in a NutriBullet(R) or blender until smooth and creamy.

Nutritional Information

- Calories: 406 kcal 20%
- Fat: 20.6 g 32%
- Carbs: 56.2g 18%

- Protein: 5.2 g 10%
- Cholesterol: 0 mg 0%
- Sodium: 172 mg 7%

Blueberry and Spice Smoothie

Ingredients
- 1/4 cup ice cubes, or as desired
- 1 cup low-fat vanilla yogurt
- 1 cup low-fat milk
- 1/2 cup frozen blueberries, or to taste
- 1 teaspoon ground cinnamon
- 1 tablespoon white sugar, or to taste
- Add all ingredients to list

Directions
1. Blend ice in a blender until crumbly; add yogurt, milk, blueberries, and cinnamon. Blend until smooth. Taste smoothie and add desired amount of sugar; blend.

Nutritional Information
- Calories: 213 kcal 11%
- Fat: 4.1 g 6%
- Carbs: 35g 11%
- Protein: 10.4 g 21%
- Cholesterol: 16 mg 5%
- Sodium: 132 mg 5%

Blueberry Banana and Peanut Butter Smoothie

"This is the perfect smoothie to get your day moving, to give you a boost, or to serve as a kid-friendly snack! "
Serving: *10 m* | **Total Time:** *10 m*

Ingredients
- 1 tablespoon flax seed meal or wheat germ
- 1 banana
- 1/2 cup frozen blueberries

- 1 tablespoon peanut butter
- 1 teaspoon honey
- 1/2 cup plain yogurt
- 1 cup milk
- Add all ingredients to list

Directions

1. Put ground flax seed meal or wheat germ into blender to grind and further breakdown. This will also eliminate any bitterness from the flax seed.
2. Place the banana, blueberries, peanut butter, honey, yogurt, and milk into the blender. Cover, and puree until smooth. Pour into glasses to serve.

Nutritional Information

- Calories: 251 kcal 13%
- Fat: 9.2 g 14%
- Carbs: 34.4g 11%
- Protein: 10.8 g 22%
- Cholesterol: 13 mg 4%
- Sodium: 132 mg 5%

Blueberry Banana Oatmeal Smoothie

"This is a quick and healthy breakfast or snack. You can easily replace the blueberries with any other fruit or berry. I've also just used banana and added some peanut butter. Yum. You can replace the sugar with Splenda®, if desired."
Serving: *10 m* | **Total Time:** *10 m*

Ingredients

- 1 cup soy milk
- 1 frozen banana, sliced
- 1/4 cup frozen blueberries
- 1/4 cup oats
- 1 tablespoon chia seeds
- 1 teaspoon vanilla extract
- 1 teaspoon white sugar, or more to taste
- Add all ingredients to list

Directions
1. Blend soy milk, banana, blueberries, oats, chia seeds, vanilla extract, and white sugar together in a blender until smooth.

Nutritional Information
- Calories: 398 kcal 20%
- Fat: 8.5 g 13%
- Carbs: 68.6g 22%
- Protein: 13.2 g 26%
- Cholesterol: 0 mg 0%
- Sodium: 129 mg 5%

Blueberry Chestnut Coconut Smoothie

Ingredients
- 4 egg yolks
- 1/2 cup frozen blueberries
- 1/2 cup coconut water
- 1/4 cup chestnut puree
- Add all ingredients to list

Directions
1. Place egg yolks, blueberries, coconut water, and chestnut puree in a blender; blend until smooth, 2 to 3 minutes.

Nutritional Information
- Calories: 313 kcal 16%
- Fat: 18.4 g 28%
- Carbs: 25.3g 8%
- Protein: 12.2 g 24%
- Cholesterol: 819 mg 273%
- Sodium: 159 mg 6%

Blueberry Cream Slushy

"My husband and I went crazy over a blueberry smoothie at a local cafe. This was our attempt to recreate it...but we actually like it better than the original!"

Serving: 5 m | Total Time: 5 m

Ingredients

- 1 cup frozen blueberries
- 1 cup frozen strawberries
- 1 cup pineapple and orange juice blend
- 1 cup vanilla yogurt
- 2 teaspoons sugar
- 6 ice cubes
- Add all ingredients to list

Directions

1. Place the blueberries, strawberries, juice, yogurt and sugar into the container of a blender. Process until smooth. Add the ice cubes, and process until small enough to fit through a straw, but large enough to crunch on. Pour into glasses, and drink through straws.

Nutritional Information

- Calories: 261 kcal 13%
- Fat: 2.1 g 3%
- Carbs: 56.2g 18%
- Protein: 6.8 g 14%
- Cholesterol: 6 mg 2%
- Sodium: 98 mg 4%

Blueberry Cucumber Smoothie

Ingredients

- 1 frozen banana, cut into chunks
- 1/2 cucumber - peeled, seeded, and cut into chunks
- 3/4 cup buttermilk
- 1/4 cup coconut water
- 2 tablespoons blueberry preserves
- Add all ingredients to list

Directions

1. Blend banana, cucumber, buttermilk, coconut water, and blueberry preserves together in a blender until smooth.

Nutritional Information
- Calories: 252 kcal 13%
- Fat: 2.3 g 4%
- Carbs: 53.5g 17%
- Protein: 8.4 g 17%
- Cholesterol: 7 mg 2%
- Sodium: 264 mg 11%

Blueberry Mango Smoothie

Ingredients
- 1 tablespoon chia seeds
- 1 (6 ounce) container vanilla yogurt
- 1/2 cup mango juice
- 1/4 cup fresh blueberries
- 1/4 cup fresh mango chunks
- 1/2 teaspoon vanilla extract
- Add all ingredients to list

Directions
1. Grind chia seeds in a food processor until pulverized; add yogurt, mango juice, blueberries, mango, and vanilla extract and blend until smooth.

Nutritional Information
- Calories: 271 kcal 14%
- Fat: 2.5 g 4%
- Carbs: 54.9g 18%
- Protein: 9.1 g 18%
- Cholesterol: 8 mg 3%
- Sodium: 117 mg 5%

Blueberry Mint Smoothie

"Vegan, gluten-free, and nut-free!"
Serving: *10 m* | **Total Time:** *10 m*

Ingredients
- 2 cups frozen blueberries

- 1 cup water
- 1 cup fresh mint leaves
- 1 avocado, peeled and pitted
- 1/2 cup orange juice
- 2 teaspoons lemon juice
- Add all ingredients to list

Directions
1. Blend blueberries, water, mint leaves, avocado, orange juice, and lemon juice in a blender until smooth.

Nutritional Information
- Calories: 273 kcal 14%
- Fat: 15.9 g 25%
- Carbs: 35g 11%
- Protein: 3.5 g 7%
- Cholesterol: 0 mg 0%
- Sodium: 13 mg < 1%

Blueberry Muffin Smoothie Shake

Ingredients
- 1/2 cup whole milk
- 1/2 cup half-and-half cream
- 2 tablespoons white sugar (optional)
- 2 teaspoons lemon extract
- 1/2 teaspoon ground cinnamon (optional)
- 1 cup frozen blueberries
- 12 vanilla wafers
- ice cubes as desired
- Add all ingredients to list

Directions
1. Blend milk, half-and-half, sugar, lemon extract, and cinnamon in a blender; add blueberries and blend until thick and smooth. Blend vanilla wafers and ice cubes into milk mixture until desired consistency is reached.

Nutritional Information
- Calories: 193 kcal 10%
- Fat: 8.2 g 13%

- Carbs: 26.7g 9%
- Protein: 2.8 g 6%
- Cholesterol: 14 mg 5%
- Sodium: 81 mg 3%

Blueberry Smoothie Bowl

Ingredients
- Smoothie:
- 1 cup frozen blueberries
- 1/2 banana
- 2 tablespoons water
- 1 tablespoon cashew butter
- 1 teaspoon vanilla extract
- Toppings:
- 1/2 banana, sliced
- 1 tablespoon sliced almonds
- 1 tablespoon unsweetened shredded coconut
- Add all ingredients to list

Directions
1. Blend blueberries, 1/2 banana, water, cashew butter, and vanilla extract together in a blender until smooth; pour into a bowl.
2. Top smoothie with sliced banana, almonds, and coconut.

Nutritional Information
- Calories: 368 kcal 18%
- Fat: 15.6 g 24%
- Carbs: 55.4g 18%
- Protein: 6.8 g 14%
- Cholesterol: 0 mg 0%
- Sodium: 8 mg < 1%

Blueberry Smoothie

"A delicious way to use up your blueberries!"
Serving: *5 m |* **Total Time:** *5 m*

Ingredients

- 1 cup blueberries (frozen or fresh)
- 1 (8 ounce) container plain yogurt
- 3/4 cup 2% reduced-fat milk
- 2 tablespoons white sugar
- 1/2 teaspoon vanilla extract
- 1/8 teaspoon ground nutmeg
- Add all ingredients to list

Directions

1. Blend the blueberries, yogurt, milk, sugar, vanilla, and nutmeg in a blender until frothy, scraping down the sides of the blender with a spatula occasionally. Serve immediately.

Nutritional Information

- Calories: 211 kcal 11%
- Fat: 3.9 g 6%
- Carbs: 35.5g 11%
- Protein: 9.5 g 19%
- Cholesterol: 14 mg 5%
- Sodium: 118 mg 5%

Blueberry Smoothies

"Try refreshing Blueberry Smoothies from Ocean Spray for a treat the whole family can enjoy all summer long."
Serving: *5 m |* **Total Time:** *5 m*

Ingredients

- 1 1/4 cups Ocean Spray® Blueberry Juice Cocktail, chilled
- 3/4 cup Ocean Spray® Fresh Blueberries, cleaned and rinsed
- 1 cup vanilla yogurt or vanilla frozen yogurt
- Add all ingredients to list

Directions

1. Combine blueberry juice cocktail and blueberries in a blender.
2. Cover; blend on high speed until mixture is smooth.
3. Add yogurt; blend until thoroughly combined.

Nutritional Information
- Calories: 205 kcal 10%
- Fat: 1.5 g 2%
- Carbs: 42.3g 14%
- Protein: 6.4 g 13%
- Cholesterol: 6 mg 2%
- Sodium: 103 mg 4%

Blueberry Spinach Protein Smoothie

Ingredients
- 1/2 pint fresh blueberries
- 2 cups fresh spinach
- 1 scoop chocolate-flavored protein powder
- Add all ingredients to list

Directions
1. Combine blueberries, spinach, and protein powder in a blender; blend until smooth.

Nutritional Information
- Calories: 183 kcal 9%
- Fat: 1.8 g 3%
- Carbs: 29.6g 10%
- Protein: 15.9 g 32%
- Cholesterol: 40 mg 13%
- Sodium: 134 mg 5%

Blueberry Vanilla Graham Protein Smoothie

Ingredients
- 1 cup coconut water, or to taste
- 1 banana, frozen
- 3/4 cup fresh blueberries
- 1/4 cup kale (optional)
- 1/4 cup spinach (optional)
- 2 medjool dates, pitted and chopped
- 1 tablespoon almond butter

- 1 tablespoon hemp seed hearts
- 1 tablespoon flax seeds
- 1 tablespoon oats
- 1 scoop vanilla protein powder (optional)
- 2 tablespoons graham cracker crumbs
- Add all ingredients to list

Directions

1. Combine coconut water, banana, blueberries, kale, spinach, dates, almond butter, hemp seed hearts, flax seeds, oats, and protein powder in a blender. Cover and puree until smooth. Top with graham cracker crumbs.

Nutritional Information

- Calories: 326 kcal 16%
- Fat: 10.4 g 16%
- Carbs: 37.3g 12%
- Protein: 25.1 g 50%
- Cholesterol: 6 mg 2%
- Sodium: 307 mg 12%

BlueCar Smoothie

Ingredients

- 2 cups almond milk
- 1 cup yogurt
- 1 banana
- 1/2 cup blueberries
- 2 pinches ground cardamom
- Add all ingredients to list

Directions

1. Blend almond milk, yogurt, banana, blueberries, and cardamom together in a blender until smooth.

Nutritional Information

- Calories: 435 kcal 22%
- Fat: 9.9 g 15%
- Carbs: 73.1g 24%
- Protein: 17 g 34%

- Cholesterol: 15 mg 5%
- Sodium: 493 mg 20%

Breakfast to Go Smoothie

"This is a smoothie for a hearty breakfast on the go."
Serving: *5 m* | **Total Time:** *5 m*

Ingredients
- 1 cup fat-free milk
- 1/2 cup frozen blueberries
- 1/2 cup plain fat-free Greek yogurt
- 1/4 cup old-fashioned oats
- 1 tablespoon ground flax seed
- Add all ingredients to list

Directions
1. Blend milk, blueberries, Greek yogurt, oats, and flax seed in a blender until smooth.

Nutritional Information
- Calories: 315 kcal 16%
- Fat: 5.4 g 8%
- Carbs: 43.4g 14%
- Protein: 23.8 g 48%
- Cholesterol: 5 mg 2%
- Sodium: 191 mg 8%

Chocolate and Blueberry Smoothie

"Refreshing and perfect for warm summer days! Kids will love this."
Serving: *5 m* | **Total Time:** *5 m*

Ingredients
- 2 teaspoons cocoa powder
- 1 teaspoon hot water
- 1 cup milk

- 4 tablespoons frozen blueberries
- 1 teaspoon white sugar
- 4 ice cubes
- Add all ingredients to list

Directions

1. Mix together the cocoa powder and water in a small bowl until the cocoa is dissolved.
2. Place the cocoa mixture, milk, blueberries, sugar, and ice cubes into a blender; cover and blend until smooth, 30 to 45 seconds. Serve cold.

Nutritional Information

- Calories: 181 kcal 9%
- Fat: 5.5 g 8%
- Carbs: 26.3g 8%
- Protein: 9.2 g 18%
- Cholesterol: 20 mg 7%
- Sodium: 104 mg 4%

Chocolate Covered Blueberry Smoothie

"This is a delicious smoothie that reminds me of the chocolate covered blueberries we bought every Christmas. Light and sweet, perfect for a summer night snack! I use fat free cocoa mix to make it lighter, or my favorite flavored cocoa mix, like chocolate hazelnut, to change it up a bit."
***Serving:** 5 m | **Total Time:** 5 m*

Ingredients

- 1 cup skim milk
- 1 cup frozen blueberries
- 1 (1 ounce) envelope instant hot chocolate mix
- 1 tablespoon chocolate syrup
- Add all ingredients to list

Directions

1. Pour the milk, blueberries, hot cocoa mix, and chocolate syrup into the container of a blender. Blend to desired consistency, and pour into a tall glass.

Nutritional Information

- Calories: 326 kcal 16%

- Fat: 2.5 g 4%
- Carbs: 66.7g 22%
- Protein: 11.2 g 22%
- Cholesterol: 5 mg 2%
- Sodium: 259 mg 10%

Daily Shake

Ingredients
- 1/2 cup Greek yogurt
- 1/2 cup almond milk
- 1/4 cup fresh spinach
- 1/4 cup fresh blueberries
- 1 tablespoon grapeseed oil
- 1 tablespoon ground chia seeds
- 1 tablespoon ground flax seed
- 1 tablespoon ground almonds
- Add all ingredients to list

Directions
1. Blend yogurt, almond milk, spinach, blueberries, grapeseed oil, chia seeds, flax seed, and almonds together in a blender until smooth.

Nutritional Information
- Calories: 408 kcal 20%
- Fat: 31.6 g 49%
- Carbs: 21.1g 7%
- Protein: 12.3 g 25%
- Cholesterol: 22 mg 8%
- Sodium: 155 mg 6%

Delicious Blueberry Smoothie

"This is a fruity, delicious, and easy-to-make smoothie."
Serving: *5 m |* **Total Time:** *5 m*

Ingredients
- 1/4 cup apple juice

- 1 tablespoon instant iced tea powder
- 1/2 cup frozen blueberries
- 1 frozen banana
- 1 tablespoon lemon juice (optional)
- Add all ingredients to list

Directions

1. Place the apple juice, iced tea powder, blueberries, banana, and lemon juice into a blender pitcher. Blend on high until smooth.

Nutritional Information

- Calories: 184 kcal 9%
- Fat: 1 g 1%
- Carbs: 46.2g 15%
- Protein: 2.1 g 4%
- Cholesterol: 0 mg 0%
- Sodium: 5 mg < 1%

Dreamy Cashew Butter Smoothie with Banana Berry Dates and Flax

Ingredients

- 1 ripe banana
- 1/2 cup cold unsweetened almond milk
- 1/3 cup frozen blueberries
- 2 dates, pitted and chopped, or more taste
- 1 1/2 tablespoons flax seeds
- 1 tablespoon cashew butter, or more to taste
- Add all ingredients to list

Directions

1. Blend banana, almond milk, blueberries, dates, flax seeds, and cashew butter together in a blender on high speed until smooth.

Nutritional Information

- Calories: 400 kcal 20%
- Fat: 17.6 g 27%
- Carbs: 59.6g 19%
- Protein: 8.5 g 17%

- Cholesterol: 0 mg 0%
- Sodium: 90 mg 4%

Frozen Berry Smoothie

Ingredients
- 1 cup milk
- 1 cup frozen berries (marionberries, raspberries, and blueberries)
- 2 tablespoons dark brown sugar
- 2 tablespoons white grape juice
- 1 teaspoon vanilla extract
- 1 ice cube
- Add all ingredients to list

Directions
1. Combine milk, berries, brown sugar, grape juice, vanilla extract, and ice cube in a blender; blend until smooth.

Nutritional Information
- Calories: 317 kcal 16%
- Fat: 5.3 g 8%
- Carbs: 60.3g 19%
- Protein: 9.3 g 19%
- Cholesterol: 20 mg 7%
- Sodium: 110 mg 4%

Frozen Blueberry Smoothie

Ingredients
- 1 cup frozen blueberries
- 3/4 cup milk
- 3/4 cup Greek yogurt
- 1 kiwi, peeled
- 2 teaspoons raw sugar
- Add all ingredients to list

Directions

1. Blend blueberries, milk, yogurt, kiwi, and sugar together in a blender until smooth.

Nutritional Information

- Calories: 443 kcal 22%
- Fat: 20 g 31%
- Carbs: 52.5g 17%
- Protein: 16.6 g 33%
- Cholesterol: 48 mg 16%
- Sodium: 180 mg 7%

Fruit Smoothie II

"A fruit smoothie that is very easy and fast. This drink is thick and good."
Serving: *5 m* | **Total Time:** *5 m*

Ingredients

- 1 cup blueberries
- 2 apples - peeled, cored and chopped
- 1 1/2 cups raspberries
- 3/4 cup seedless grapes
- 3 tablespoons white sugar
- 1 tray ice cubes
- Add all ingredients to list

Directions

1. In a blender, combine blueberries, apples, raspberries, grapes, sugar and ice. Blend until smooth. Pour into glasses and serve.

Nutritional Information

- Calories: 137 kcal 7%
- Fat: 0.7 g 1%
- Carbs: 34.8g 11%
- Protein: 1.1 g 2%
- Cholesterol: 0 mg 0%
- Sodium: 4 mg < 1%

Fruity 3 Step Acai Bowl Healthy ICE cream!

Ingredients

- 1 banana, broken into chunks
- 1/2 cup almond milk
- 6 fresh blackberries, divided
- 6 hulled strawberries, divided
- 2 ice cubes
- 1 tablespoon coconut yogurt
- 1 1/2 teaspoons acai powder
- 1/2 mango, peeled and chopped, or more to taste
- 1/2 cup granola
- 2 tablespoons shredded coconut, or more to taste
- 2 tablespoons blueberries, or more to taste
- 1 tablespoon almond butter, or to taste
- 1 teaspoon honey, or as desired
- Add all ingredients to list

Directions

1. Blend banana, almond milk, 3 blackberries, 4 strawberries, ice cubes, coconut yogurt, and acai powder in a blender until smooth; pour into a bowl. Top mixture with mango, granola, coconut, 3 blackberries, 4 strawberries, blueberries, almond butter, and honey.

Nutritional Information

- Calories: 780 kcal 39%
- Fat: 36.2 g 56%
- Carbs: 106.8g 34%
- Protein: 15.9 g 32%
- Cholesterol: 0 mg 0%
- Sodium: 178 mg 7%

Ginger Berry Smoothie

Ingredients

- 1 cup water, or more as needed
- 1/4 cup frozen blueberries
- 4 frozen strawberries, or more to taste
- 1 (1 inch) piece fresh ginger, peeled and coarsely chopped
- 1 tablespoon agave nectar

- Add all ingredients to list

Directions

1. Blend water, blueberries, strawberries, ginger, and agave nectar together in a blender until thick and smooth.

Nutritional Information

- Calories: 103 kcal 5%
- Fat: 0.3 g < 1%
- Carbs: 26.8g 9%
- Protein: 0.7 g 1%
- Cholesterol: 0 mg 0%
- Sodium: 9 mg < 1%

Ginger Fruit Smoothie

Ingredients

- 1 cup water, or more as needed
- 1/4 cup frozen blueberries
- 1/4 cup seedless green grapes
- 1/2 green apple, cored and chopped
- 3 frozen strawberries, or more to taste
- 1 (1 inch) piece peeled fresh ginger, cut into thirds
- 1 tablespoon agave nectar
- Add all ingredients to list

Directions

1. Blend water, blueberries, grapes, apple, strawberries, ginger, and agave nectar together in a blender until thick and slushy.

Nutritional Information

- Calories: 164 kcal 8%
- Fat: 0.6 g < 1%
- Carbs: 42.5g 14%
- Protein: 1.1 g 2%
- Cholesterol: 0 mg 0%
- Sodium: 10 mg < 1%

Gordon's Berry Breakfast Drink

"I like to serve this drink in my cobalt blue glasses. It's tasty and colorful!"
Serving: *5 m* | **Total Time:** *5 m*

Ingredients
- 3/4 cup chilled orange juice
- 1/3 cup chilled pineapple juice
- 2 cups vanilla yogurt
- 1 cup frozen blueberries
- 1/2 cup frozen sliced strawberries
- 1/2 banana, sliced
- Add all ingredients to list

Directions
1. Place the orange juice, pineapple juice, yogurt, blueberries, strawberries, and bananas into a blender. Cover and blend until smooth. The berry drink will be very thick. Serve immediately.

Nutritional Information
- Calories: 120 kcal 6%
- Fat: 1.2 g 2%
- Carbs: 23.7g 8%
- Protein: 4.7 g 9%
- Cholesterol: 4 mg 1%
- Sodium: 55 mg 2%

Green Drink with Aloe Vera Juice

Ingredients
- 1 cup aloe vera juice
- 1/2 cup old-fashioned rolled oats
- 1 cup baby spinach
- 1 cup baby kale
- 1 cup baby chard
- 1 banana
- 1/2 cucumber
- 1/2 cup fresh blueberries
- 2 tablespoons protein powder (optional)

- 1 teaspoon ground cinnamon
- 1 pinch cayenne pepper
- Add all ingredients to list

Directions

1. Mix aloe vera juice and oats together in a bowl; set aside until oats have absorbed the liquid, about 10 minutes.
2. Blend oat mixture, spinach, kale, chard, banana, cucumber, blueberries, protein powder, cinnamon, and cayenne pepper together in a blender until smooth, about 2 minutes.

Nutritional Information

- Calories: 537 kcal 27%
- Fat: 5.2 g 8%
- Carbs: 107.2g 35%
- Protein: 24.3 g 49%
- Cholesterol: 0 mg 0%
- Sodium: 327 mg 13%

Green Monster Spinach Smoothie

Ingredients

- 1 cup yogurt
- 1 banana, broken into chunks
- 1/2 cup frozen blueberries
- 4 cups fresh spinach
- 1 tablespoon water, or as desired (optional)
- 2 ice cubes, or as desired (optional)
- Add all ingredients to list

Directions

1. Layer yogurt, banana, and blueberries in a blender, respectively. Add as much spinach to blender that will fit; pour in water. Blend on high speed until smooth, adding the remaining spinach if needed. Add ice for a colder and thicker smoothie. Add more water for a thinner smoothie.

Nutritional Information

- Calories: 164 kcal 8%
- Fat: 2.4 g 4%
- Carbs: 29.5g 10%

- Protein: 9.1 g 18%
- Cholesterol: 7 mg 2%
- Sodium: 135 mg 5%

Green Smoothie Bowl

Ingredients
- Smoothie:
- 3 cups fresh spinach
- 1 banana
- 1/2 (14 ounce) can coconut milk
- 1/2 cup frozen mango chunks
- 1/2 cup coconut water
- Toppings:
- 1/3 cup fresh raspberries
- 1/4 cup fresh blueberries
- 2 tablespoons granola
- 1 tablespoon coconut flakes
- 1/4 teaspoon sliced almonds
- 1/4 teaspoon chia seeds (optional)
- Add all ingredients to list

Directions
1. Blend spinach, banana, coconut milk, mango, and coconut water in a blender until smooth. Pour smoothie into a bowl and top with raspberries, blueberries, granola, coconut flakes, almonds, and chia seeds.

Nutritional Information
- Calories: 374 kcal 19%
- Fat: 25.6 g 39%
- Carbs: 37g 12%
- Protein: 6.3 g 13%
- Cholesterol: 0 mg 0%
- Sodium: 116 mg 5%

Hailey's Smoothie

"A healthy drink with kiwis, bananas, blueberries and yogurt. Quick and satisfying for breakfast or any time of day!"
Serving: *2 m* | **Total Time:** *2 m*

Ingredients
- 3 kiwis, peeled and chopped
- 2 frozen bananas, peeled and chopped
- 1 cup blueberries
- 1 cup plain yogurt
- 1 1/2 cups crushed ice
- 3 tablespoons honey
- 1/4 teaspoon almond extract
- Add all ingredients to list

Directions
1. In a blender, combine the kiwis, frozen bananas, blueberries, yogurt, crushed ice, honey and almond extract. Blend until smooth.

Nutritional Information
- Calories: 194 kcal 10%
- Fat: 1.6 g 2%
- Carbs: 44.2g 14%
- Protein: 4.8 g 10%
- Cholesterol: 4 mg 1%
- Sodium: 47 mg 2%

Healthy Blueberry Breakfast Smoothie

"A quick recipe I thought up while trying to decide what to eat for breakfast. Great if you are trying to figure out what to do with those blueberries in the fridge or freezer! Also great on-the-go! Delicious and includes many foods that are a great way to start your day! Many of the ingredients, except for the blueberries and yogurt, are optional and vary depending on your own taste. I love cinnamon and a thick, super-cold smoothie. This recipe is super versatile, and you can change it depending on dietary needs or personal preference. Have fun with it!"
Serving: *15 m* | **Total Time:** *15 m*

Ingredients
- 1 cup fresh blueberries
- 1/2 cup Greek yogurt
- 1/4 cup orange juice
- 1 tablespoon white sugar, or to taste
- 1/4 teaspoon vanilla extract
- 1 pinch ground cinnamon, or to taste
- 3 ice cubes
- Add all ingredients to list

Directions
1. Blend blueberries, yogurt, orange juice, sugar, vanilla extract, and cinnamon together in a blender on low speed for 30 seconds; increase speed to high and blend until smooth, about 2 minutes. Add ice and blend on high until smooth, about 1 minute more.

Nutritional Information
- Calories: 295 kcal 15%
- Fat: 10.6 g 16%
- Carbs: 44.9g 14%
- Protein: 7.5 g 15%
- Cholesterol: 22 mg 8%
- Sodium: 69 mg 3%

Healthy Fruit and Vegetable Smoothie

Ingredients
- 6 fluid ounces milk
- 1 (6 ounce) container plain yogurt
- 1/2 cup frozen strawberries
- 1/2 frozen banana
- 1/4 cup frozen blueberries
- 1 green ice cube (see footnote)
- 2 tablespoons whey protein powder (optional)
- 1 teaspoon honey, or to taste
- Add all ingredients to list

Directions
1. Combine milk, yogurt, strawberries, banana, blueberries, green ice cube, whey, and honey in a blender, in the order listed. Blend until smooth.

Nutritional Information
- Calories: 372 kcal 19%
- Fat: 6.8 g 10%
- Carbs: 63.2g 20%
- Protein: 18.1 g 36%
- Cholesterol: 26 mg 9%
- Sodium: 358 mg 14%

Heart Healthy Blueberry Smoothie

"This is a fantastic smoothie if you're searching for something that is heart-healthy and antioxidant-rich!"
***Serving:** 10 m | **Total Time:** 10 m*

Ingredients
- 1 cup blueberries
- 3/4 cup pomegranate juice
- 1/2 cup low-fat plain Greek-style yogurt
- 1/2 cup skim milk
- 1/2 cup rolled oats
- 1/4 cup granular sucralose sweetener (such as Splenda®)
- 1 teaspoon ground cinnamon
- Add all ingredients to list

Directions
1. Blend blueberries, pomegranate juice, yogurt, milk, oats, sweetener, and cinnamon together in a blender until smooth, about 2 minutes.

Nutritional Information
- Calories: 252 kcal 13%
- Fat: 2.8 g 4%
- Carbs: 53.3g 17%
- Protein: 10.1 g 20%
- Cholesterol: 4 mg 1%
- Sodium: 50 mg 2%

Heavenly Blueberry Smoothie

"This blueberry smoothie is to die for! It tastes so good, you forget that it's good for ya!"
Serving: *10 m |* **Total Time:** *10 m*

Ingredients
- 1 frozen banana, thawed for 10 to 15 minutes
- 1/2 cup vanilla soy milk
- 1 cup vanilla fat-free yogurt
- 1 1/2 teaspoons flax seed meal
- 1 1/2 teaspoons honey
- 2/3 cup frozen blueberries
- Add all ingredients to list

Directions
1. Cut banana into small pieces and place into the bowl of a blender. Add the soy milk, yogurt, flax seed meal, and honey. Blend on lowest speed until smooth, about 5 seconds. Gradually add the blueberries while continuing to blend on low. Once the blueberries have been incorporated, increase speed, and blend to desired consistency.

Nutritional Information
- Calories: 250 kcal 13%
- Fat: 2.6 g 4%
- Carbs: 50.2g 16%
- Protein: 9.5 g 19%
- Cholesterol: 2 mg < 1%
- Sodium: 117 mg 5%

Kids' Choice Healthilicious Pineapple Smoothie

"This is my kids' favorite smoothie! The main flavors of this smoothie are pineapple and vanilla but it is full of antioxidants from berries and spinach! Great way to get your greens."
Serving: *10 m |* **Total Time:** *10 m*

Ingredients

- 8 ounces vanilla fat-free yogurt
- 2 1/2 ounces baby spinach leaves
- 1 cup fresh blueberries
- 1/2 cup frozen pineapple chunks
- 1/2 cup fresh raspberries
- 1/4 cup water
- 1 cup crushed ice
- Add all ingredients to list

Directions

1. Blend yogurt and baby spinach together in a blender until spinach is finely chopped. Add blueberries, pineapple, raspberries, and water; blend until smooth. Add crushed ice and blend again until smooth.

Nutritional Information

- Calories: 110 kcal 5%
- Fat: 0.4 g < 1%
- Carbs: 24.3g 8%
- Protein: 3.9 g 8%
- Cholesterol: < 1 mg < 1%
- Sodium: 55 mg 2%

Marlene's Yogurt Berry Smoothie

Ingredients

- 1 cup soy milk
- 2 tablespoons flax seed meal
- 1 cup Greek yogurt (such as Chobani®)
- 1 cup fresh strawberries
- 1/2 banana
- 3 ounces baby carrots, cut into chunks
- 1 tablespoon flaked coconut
- 1 cup frozen blueberries
- Add all ingredients to list

Directions

1. Pour soy milk and flax seeds into a blender. Allow flax seeds to soften, 1 to 3 minutes. Turn blender on and add yogurt, strawberries, banana, carrots, and coconut, blending well after each addition. Add blueberries and blend until

smooth.

Nutritional Information
- Calories: 359 kcal 18%
- Fat: 17.6 g 27%
- Carbs: 41g 13%
- Protein: 13.1 g 26%
- Cholesterol: 22 mg 8%
- Sodium: 165 mg 7%

Morning Energy Booster Smoothie

Ingredients
- 1 cup prune juice
- 3 tablespoons vanilla Greek yogurt
- 1 cup fresh spinach, or to taste
- 1 cup frozen blueberries, or to taste
- 6 frozen strawberries
- 1/2 sliced frozen peach
- 2 tablespoons flax seeds
- Add all ingredients to list

Directions
1. Pour prune juice into a blender. Layer Greek yogurt, spinach, blueberries, strawberries, peach, and flax seeds in the blender, in this order. Start blender on low speed and gradually increase speed until smoothie is well blended.

Nutritional Information
- Calories: 239 kcal 12%
- Fat: 5.6 g 9%
- Carbs: 44.7g 14%
- Protein: 6.1 g 12%
- Cholesterol: 1 mg < 1%
- Sodium: 33 mg 1%

Overnight Oats Blueberry Smoothie Bowl

Ingredients
- 1 cup rolled oats
- 1 1/4 cups unsweetened vanilla-flavored almond milk, divided
- 1 frozen banana, chopped
- 1 cup blueberries
- 1 teaspoon vanilla extract
- 1 teaspoon maple syrup, or to taste
- Topping:
- 2 tablespoons flaked coconut
- 1 tablespoon fresh blueberries
- 1 teaspoon chia seeds
- Add all ingredients to list

Directions
1. Combine oats and 2/3 cup almond milk in a bowl; refrigerate until oats have absorbed the liquid, 8 hours to overnight.
2. Combine oats-almond milk mixture, remaining almond milk, banana, 1 cup blueberries, vanilla extract, and maple syrup in a blender; blend until smooth.
3. Pour smoothie into 2 bowls and top with coconut, 1 tablespoon blueberries, and chia seeds.

Nutritional Information
- Calories: 354 kcal 18%
- Fat: 6.5 g 10%
- Carbs: 68.7g 22%
- Protein: 7.6 g 15%
- Cholesterol: 0 mg 0%
- Sodium: 118 mg 5%

Penny's Smoothie

"Banana, blueberries and peaches blended with yogurt and fruit syrup. Use any flavor of syrup to taste. My kids like to freeze this for ice pops."
Serving: *10 m |* **Total Time:** *10 m*

Ingredients
- 1 banana

- 1/4 cup frozen blueberries
- 3/4 cup frozen peach slices
- 1/4 cup yogurt
- 2 tablespoons all fruit blueberry syrup
- 1/8 cup rice milk
- Add all ingredients to list

Directions

1. In a blender, combine banana, frozen blueberries, frozen peach slices, yogurt and syrup. Blend until smooth. add rice milk and blend to desired consistency. Pour into glasses and serve.

Nutritional Information

- Calories: 139 kcal 7%
- Fat: 0.7 g 1%
- Carbs: 33.1g 11%
- Protein: 2.1 g 4%
- Cholesterol: 1 mg < 1%
- Sodium: 24 mg < 1%

Prairie Berry Smoothie

Ingredients

- 3/4 cup milk
- 1/4 cup frozen blueberries
- 1/4 cup frozen raspberries
- 1/4 cup frozen mango chunks
- 2 tablespoons vanilla yogurt, or more to taste
- 1 banana
- Add all ingredients to list

Directions

1. Blend milk, blueberries, raspberries, mango, and yogurt together in a blender until smooth. Add banana and blend until smooth.

Nutritional Information

- Calories: 338 kcal 17%
- Fat: 4.8 g 7%
- Carbs: 69g 22%

- Protein: 9.9 g 20%
- Cholesterol: 16 mg 5%
- Sodium: 98 mg 4%

Pre Packaged Smoothies

"Ready-made smoothies are frozen in plastic bags, all ready to be blended."
Serving: 4 h 15 m | Total Time: 4 h 15 m

Ingredients
- 4 (8 ounce) containers plain lowfat yogurt
- 2 cups sliced fresh strawberries
- 2 cups fresh blueberries
- 2 bananas, halved
- Add all ingredients to list

Directions
1. Transfer each container of yogurt into a muffin cup and freeze solid, about 4 hours. Remove frozen yogurt; place 1 portion of frozen yogurt into a resealable plastic bag and add 1/2 cup strawberries, 1/2 cup blueberries, and half a banana to each bag. Store the bags in the freezer until serving time. Place contents of a bag into a blender and blend until smooth.

Nutritional Information
- Calories: 263 kcal 13%
- Fat: 4.2 g 6%
- Carbs: 46.3g 15%
- Protein: 13.7 g 27%
- Cholesterol: 14 mg 5%
- Sodium: 161 mg 6%

Purple Monstrosity Fruit Smoothie

"This is a great smoothie for breakfast - and sometimes dinner! You can substitute the orange juice with any mix of juices or even soy milk! The soy milk adds more of a milk shake quality than the juice does."
Serving: 5 m | Total Time: 5 m

Ingredients

- 2 frozen bananas, skins removed and cut in chunks
- 1/2 cup frozen blueberries
- 1 cup orange juice
- 1 tablespoon honey (optional)
- 1 teaspoon vanilla extract (optional)
- Add all ingredients to list

Directions

1. Place bananas, blueberries and juice in a blender, puree. Use honey and/or vanilla to taste. Use more or less liquid depending on the thickness you want for your smoothie.

Nutritional Information

- Calories: 87 kcal 4%
- Fat: 0.4 g < 1%
- Carbs: 21.4g 7%
- Protein: 0.9 g 2%
- Cholesterol: 0 mg 0%
- Sodium: 1 mg < 1%

Purple Moose Canadian Smoothie

Ingredients

- 15 ice cubes
- 1 ripe banana
- 1/2 cup vanilla rice milk
- 1/4 cup fresh blueberries
- 2 tablespoons natural peanut butter
- 2 tablespoons maple syrup
- Add all ingredients to list

Directions

1. Combine ice cubes, banana, rice milk, blueberries, peanut butter, and maple syrup in a blender; blend on low speed. Increase speed to medium-high and blend until smooth.

Nutritional Information

- Calories: 241 kcal 12%
- Fat: 8.7 g 13%

- Carbs: 39.9g 13%
- Protein: 4.9 g 10%
- Cholesterol: 0 mg 0%
- Sodium: 70 mg 3%

Purple Power Punch Smoothie My Kids' Fave

"This is my go-to smoothie of choice. My kids (all 4) absolutely love it for the flavor as well as the purple color. It's fun, easy, and the kids can even help out! Feel free to add or subtract any of the fruit, honey, or sugar to your taste preference."
Serving: *10 m* | **Total Time:** *10 m*

Ingredients
- 1/2 cup nonfat vanilla yogurt (such as Dannon® Light and Fit®)
- 1/2 cup sliced strawberries
- 1/2 cup water
- 1/2 cup nonfat powdered milk
- 1 banana, cut in chunks
- 1/4 cup blueberries, or to taste
- 1/4 cup raspberries, or to taste
- 1/4 cup blackberries, or to taste
- 2 scoops vanilla whey protein powder
- 1 cup crushed ice
- 3 tablespoons turbinado sugar (such as Sugar in the Raw®)
- 1 tablespoon honey
- Add all ingredients to list

Directions
1. Pulse yogurt, strawberries, water, powdered milk, banana, blueberries, raspberries, blackberries, and protein powder together in a blender until well-mixed. Add ice, sugar, and honey and blend until smooth.

Nutritional Information
- Calories: 177 kcal 9%
- Fat: 0.7 g 1%
- Carbs: 26.5g 9%
- Protein: 17.7 g 35%
- Cholesterol: 6 mg 2%
- Sodium: 142 mg 6%

Rainier Cherry Berry Smoothie

Ingredients
- 1 banana
- 3/4 cup blueberries
- 1/2 cup fat-free vanilla yogurt
- 6 large fresh strawberries, halved
- 12 Rainier cherries, pitted and halved
- 1/4 cup fat-free milk
- Add all ingredients to list

Directions
1. Combine banana, blueberries, vanilla yogurt, strawberries, cherries, and milk in a blender; blend until smooth, about 60 seconds.

Nutritional Information
- Calories: 199 kcal 10%
- Fat: 1.1 g 2%
- Carbs: 44.7g 14%
- Protein: 6.3 g 13%
- Cholesterol: 2 mg < 1%
- Sodium: 62 mg 2%

Razzy Blue Smoothie

"This naturally sweet and creamy, frosty cold smoothie packs a lot of flavor and a nutritious punch."
Serving: *10 m* | **Total Time:** *10 m*

Ingredients
- 1 banana
- 16 whole almonds
- 1/4 cup rolled oats
- 1 tablespoon flaxseed meal
- 1 cup frozen blueberries
- 1 cup raspberry yogurt
- 1/4 cup Concord grape juice
- 1 cup 1% buttermilk

- Add all ingredients to list

Directions

1. Peel the banana and cut into 1/2-inch chunks. Chill in freezer until solid, about 2 hours.
2. Place the almonds, oats, and flaxseed meal into a blender; pulse until finely ground. Add the frozen banana, frozen blueberries, yogurt, grape juice, and buttermilk; puree until smooth.

Nutritional Information

- Calories: 262 kcal 13%
- Fat: 6.5 g 10%
- Carbs: 44.5g 14%
- Protein: 8.8 g 18%
- Cholesterol: 8 mg 3%
- Sodium: 142 mg 6%

Red White and Blue Fruit Smoothie

"This delicious smoothie is sweetened with natural sugars. Replace any of the fruit ingredients with your favorites if you like, but make sure one of them is frozen to make it nice and thick!"
***Serving:** 5 m | **Total Time:** 5 m*

Ingredients

- 1/2 large banana, cut into pieces and frozen
- 2 large fresh strawberries, rinsed and sliced
- 1/4 cup blueberries
- 1/2 cup milk
- 1 teaspoon vanilla extract
- 2 tablespoons vanilla yogurt
- 2 ice cubes
- Add all ingredients to list

Directions

1. Place the banana pieces, strawberries, blueberries, milk, vanilla extract, yogurt, and ice cubes in a blender. Blend until smooth.

Nutritional Information

- Calories: 192 kcal 10%

- Fat: 3.2 g 5%
- Carbs: 34g 11%
- Protein: 6.8 g 14%
- Cholesterol: 11 mg 4%
- Sodium: 73 mg 3%

Salad Smoothie

"Going raw is a great lifestyle choice. You can find a lot of fruit smoothies that taste good. Here is a great vegetable one too."
Serving: *10 m |* **Total Time:** *10 m*

Ingredients
- 1 cup water, or as desired
- 1/2 orange, peeled
- 1 cup fresh spinach
- 1/2 raw beet, peeled
- 1/3 cup baby carrots
- 1/3 cup cauliflower florets
- 1/3 cup broccoli florets
- 1/4 cup blueberries, or to taste
- 1 stalk celery
- 1/2 lime, peeled
- 1 tablespoon honey
- 1 tablespoon chia seeds
- Add all ingredients to list

Directions
1. Pour water into the pitcher of a high-powered blender; add the orange, spinach, beet, carrots, cauliflower, broccoli, blueberries, celery, lime, honey, and chia seeds. Blend on high speed until smooth, about 1 minute.

Nutritional Information
- Calories: 199 kcal 10%
- Fat: 3 g 5%
- Carbs: 43.6g 14%
- Protein: 5.5 g 11%
- Cholesterol: 0 mg 0%
- Sodium: 149 mg 6%

Simple Summer Smoothie

"I just gathered together my favorite fruits and added what else was needed. If you like, use a multigrain bar (I use Entenmann's strawberry flavored), crumble it, and sprinkle some on top of each smoothie."
Serving: *10 m* | **Total Time:** *10 m*

Ingredients
- 1 banana
- 1 cup frozen strawberries
- 1 cup frozen blueberries
- 1 cup frozen cherries
- 4 ice cubes
- 1/2 cup orange juice
- 3/4 cup vanilla yogurt
- 1/2 teaspoon honey (optional)
- Add all ingredients to list

Directions
1. Place the banana, strawberries, blueberries, cherries, and ice cubes into a blender. Pour in the orange juice, vanilla yogurt, and honey. Puree until smooth.

Nutritional Information
- Calories: 139 kcal 7%
- Fat: 1.2 g 2%
- Carbs: 31.1g 10%
- Protein: 3.6 g 7%
- Cholesterol: 2 mg < 1%
- Sodium: 33 mg 1%

Strawberry and Blueberry Oatmeal Health Shake

Ingredients
- 1 cup frozen blueberries
- 3/4 cup skim milk
- 5 large strawberries
- 1/2 cup white sugar
- 1/2 cup oatmeal
- 1/4 cup vanilla and honey Greek yogurt (such as Chobani®)

- 1 cup ice, or to taste
- Add all ingredients to list

Directions
1. Combine blueberries, milk, strawberries, sugar, oatmeal, and yogurt in a blender; blend until smooth. Add ice; blend until smooth.

Nutritional Information
- Calories: 371 kcal 19%
- Fat: 2.8 g 4%
- Carbs: 81.6g 26%
- Protein: 7.8 g 16%
- Cholesterol: 4 mg 1%
- Sodium: 101 mg 4%

Strawberry Blueberry Smoothies

"A delicious start to your day. If I have extra I freeze it in ice cube trays so later I can just blend the cubes, so much better than wasting leftovers. My 2-year-old daughter loves it too!"
Serving: 5 m | Total Time: 5 m

Ingredients
- 1/2 cup almond milk
- 1/2 cup frozen strawberries
- 1/2 cup frozen blueberries
- 1/2 cup low-fat plain yogurt
- 1 teaspoon flax seed oil
- 1 teaspoon agave nectar
- Add all ingredients to list

Directions
1. Blend almond milk, strawberries, blueberries, yogurt, flax seed oil, and agave nectar in a blender until smooth.

Nutritional Information
- Calories: 231 kcal 12%
- Fat: 5.3 g 8%
- Carbs: 40g 13%

- Protein: 8.7 g 17%
- Cholesterol: 7 mg 2%
- Sodium: 170 mg 7%

Summer Sweet Smoothies

"Packed full of sweet summer fruity goodness. Great for a breakfast or lunch when you're on the go."
Serving: *5 m |* **Total Time:** *5 m*

Ingredients
- 2 cups cranberry juice
- 2 cups strawberries
- 1 cup blueberries
- 1 cup watermelon chunks
- 1 banana
- 2 fresh figs
- Add all ingredients to list

Directions
1. Process the cranberry juice, strawberries, blueberries, watermelon, banana, and figs in a blender until smooth and creamy. Enjoy immediately or keep cool in refrigerator.

Nutritional Information
- Calories: 168 kcal 8%
- Fat: 0.7 g 1%
- Carbs: 42.3g 14%
- Protein: 1.5 g 3%
- Cholesterol: 0 mg 0%
- Sodium: 5 mg < 1%

Super Healthy Fruit Smoothie

"Absolutely wonderful fruit smoothie with raspberries, blueberries, strawberries and more! I have this for breakfast every morning."
Serving: *10 m |* **Total Time:** *10 m*

Ingredients

- 1/3 cup fresh blueberries
- 1/3 cup fresh raspberries
- 4 large fresh strawberries, hulled
- 1/3 cup pomegranate juice
- 1/3 cup mango juice
- 2/3 cup milk
- 2 tablespoons honey
- Add all ingredients to list

Directions

1. Place the blueberries, raspberries, strawberries, pomegranate and mango juices, milk, and honey into a blender. Cover, and puree until smooth. Pour into glasses to serve.

Nutritional Information

- Calories: 191 kcal 10%
- Fat: 1.9 g 3%
- Carbs: 42.7g 14%
- Protein: 3.4 g 7%
- Cholesterol: 7 mg 2%
- Sodium: 37 mg 1%

Super Smoothie

"This is a fun and easy recipe for summer fun."
Serving: *10 m* | **Total Time:** *10 m*

Ingredients

- 1 cup frozen blueberries
- 1/2 cup sliced banana
- 1/2 cup sliced peeled cucumber
- 1/2 cup water
- 1/2 cup vanilla yogurt
- 1/2 cup crushed ice, or as needed
- Add all ingredients to list

Directions

1. Blend blueberries, banana, cucumber, water, and yogurt together in a blender until smooth. Add crushed ice and blend until smooth.

Nutritional Information
- Calories: 64 kcal 3%
- Fat: 0.7 g 1%
- Carbs: 13.6g 4%
- Protein: 2 g 4%
- Cholesterol: 2 mg < 1%
- Sodium: 23 mg < 1%

Supercharged Breakfast Smoothie

Ingredients
- 1 1/2 cups almond milk, or as needed
- 1/2 cup rolled oats
- 1/2 cup strawberries
- 1/4 cup blueberries
- 2 clementines, peeled and segmented
- 1 apple, cored and cut into chunks
- 1/2 avocado - peeled, pitted, and diced
- 2 tablespoons flax seeds
- 1 1/2 tablespoons honey
- 1 tablespoon extra-virgin coconut oil
- 1 tablespoon chia seeds
- Add all ingredients to list

Directions
1. Blend almond milk, oats, strawberries, blueberries, clementines, apple, avocado, flax seeds, honey, coconut oil, and chia seeds together in a blender until smooth, 30 to 60 seconds.

Nutritional Information
- Calories: 491 kcal 25%
- Fat: 24.4 g 38%
- Carbs: 66.9g 22%
- Protein: 8.4 g 17%
- Cholesterol: 0 mg 0%
- Sodium: 132 mg 5%

Superfood Berry Green Smoothie

"This is a meal-sized breakfast smoothie that will fill you up from morning until lunch. High in anti-oxidants, fiber, protein, and vitamin C, this smoothie is both tasty and healthy!"
Serving: *10 m* | **Total Time:** *10 m*

Ingredients
- 1 1/4 cups unsweetened almond milk
- 1 clementine (such as Cuties®), peeled
- 1/2 cup frozen raspberries
- 1 cup spinach, or more to taste
- 1 tablespoon chia seeds
- 1 tablespoon flaxseed meal
- 1 cup frozen blueberries
- 1 scoop vanilla protein powder
- Add all ingredients to list

Directions
1. Place almond milk, clementine, raspberries, spinach, chia seeds, flaxseed meal, blueberries, and protein powder in the blender, respectively. Blend on high until smooth, about 30 seconds.

Nutritional Information
- Calories: 490 kcal 24%
- Fat: 11.5 g 18%
- Carbs: 58g 19%
- Protein: 44 g 88%
- Cholesterol: 12 mg 4%
- Sodium: 443 mg 18%

Superfood Green Smoothie

Ingredients
- 1 cup spinach leaves
- 1 cup shredded kale
- 1/2 pear, cut into chunks
- 1/2 large ripe banana, sliced
- 1/2 cup frozen blueberries
- 1/3 cup plain yogurt

- 4 ice cubes
- 2 tablespoons ground flax seeds
- 1/2 cup brewed green tea, chilled, or more to taste
- Add all ingredients to list

Directions

1. Combine spinach, kale, pear, banana, blueberries, yogurt, ice cubes, and ground flax seeds in a blender; pour in tea. Blend on high until mixture is smooth. Mix with a wooden spoon to redistribute ingredients if needed.

Nutritional Information

- Calories: 175 kcal 9%
- Fat: 6.3 g 10%
- Carbs: 27.4g 9%
- Protein: 5.9 g 12%
- Cholesterol: 2 mg < 1%
- Sodium: 54 mg 2%

Triple Threat Fruit Smoothie

"A wonderful, delightful fruit smoothie...it will help you cool down after a hot day in the sun."
Serving: 5 m | Total Time: 5 m

Ingredients

- 1 kiwi, sliced
- 1 banana, peeled and chopped
- 1/2 cup blueberries
- 1 cup strawberries
- 1 cup ice cubes
- 1/2 cup orange juice
- 1 (8 ounce) container peach yogurt
- Add all ingredients to list

Directions

1. In a blender, blend the kiwi, banana, blueberries, strawberries, ice, orange juice, and yogurt until smooth.

Nutritional Information

- Calories: 134 kcal 7%

- Fat: 1.1 g 2%
- Carbs: 29.6g 10%
- Protein: 3.6 g 7%
- Cholesterol: 4 mg 1%
- Sodium: 41 mg 2%

Very Berry Blueberry Smoothie

"If you love blueberries, this is the smoothie for you! It's quick, easy, and enjoyable! It's a definite 'Yummy in the Tummy!'"
Serving: 5 m | Total Time: 5 m

Ingredients
- 1 banana, chopped
- 1 kiwi, sliced
- 3/4 cup blueberries
- 1 cup ice cubes
- 1 (8 ounce) container vanilla yogurt
- Add all ingredients to list

Directions
1. Combine the banana, kiwi, blueberries, ice cubes, and vanilla yogurt in a blender; blend until smooth.

Nutritional Information
- Calories: 135 kcal 7%
- Fat: 1.3 g 2%
- Carbs: 28.4g 9%
- Protein: 4.7 g 9%
- Cholesterol: 4 mg 1%
- Sodium: 54 mg 2%

Very Berry Smoothie

Ingredients
- 1 1/2 cups frozen blueberries
- 1/2 cup fresh raspberries
- 1/2 cup cranberry juice
- 1/3 cup peach juice

- 1/3 cup water
- 6 ice cubes, or as desired
- Add all ingredients to list

Directions
1. Blend blueberries, raspberries, cranberry juice, peach juice, and water together in a blender until smooth. Add ice cubes to blender and blend until cubes are completely crushed, about 1 minute.

Nutritional Information
- Calories: 131 kcal 7%
- Fat: 1 g 2%
- Carbs: 32g 10%
- Protein: 0.9 g 2%
- Cholesterol: 0 mg 0%
- Sodium: 8 mg < 1%

Chapter 5: Green Smoothies

***

Ann's Berry Green Smoothie

Ingredients
- 2 cups frozen strawberries
- 1 1/2 cups warm water
- 2 cups milk
- 1 1/2 cups fresh spinach, or to taste
- 1 cup frozen blueberries
- 1 frozen chopped banana
- 1 tablespoon honey
- 1/2 lemon, juiced
- Add all ingredients to list

Directions
1. Place strawberries in a bowl; add warm water.
2. Blend milk and spinach together in a blender until smooth. Add blueberries, banana, and honey and blend until smooth. Add strawberries-water mixture and lemon juice and blend until smooth.

Nutritional Information
- Calories: 303 kcal 15%
- Fat: 5.7 g 9%
- Carbs: 57.4g 19%
- Protein: 10.3 g 21%
- Cholesterol: 20 mg 7%
- Sodium: 128 mg 5%

Antioxidant King

Ingredients
- 1/4 fresh pineapple, peeled
- 1 Golden Delicious apple, quartered
- 1 small beet, top and bottom trimmed
- 1/4 cup fresh spinach, or to taste
- 1/4 cup mixed berries, or to taste
- 1/2 banana
- 1/2 avocado, peeled
- 3 ice cubes

- Add all ingredients to list

Directions
1. Process pineapple, apple, beet, and spinach through a juicer.
2. Blend juice, berries, banana, avocado, and ice cubes in a blender until smooth.

Nutritional Information
- Calories: 485 kcal 24%
- Fat: 15.6 g 24%
- Carbs: 93.2g 30%
- Protein: 6.4 g 13%
- Cholesterol: 0 mg 0%
- Sodium: 73 mg 3%

Any Way You Want It Kale Smoothie

"My toddler loves this one and he gets a serving of each: milk, fruit, and veggie!"
***Serving:** 10 m | **Total Time:** 10 m*

Ingredients
- 2 cups chopped kale
- 1/4 cup Greek yogurt
- 3 tablespoons peanuts (optional)
- 1/2 cup milk
- 1/2 frozen banana
- 3 frozen strawberries, or more to taste
- 1 tablespoon maple syrup
- Add all ingredients to list

Directions
1. Blend kale, yogurt, and peanuts together in a blender until smooth. Add milk, banana, strawberries, and maple syrup and blend until desired consistency is reached.

Nutritional Information
- Calories: 469 kcal 23%
- Fat: 22.2 g 34%
- Carbs: 56.8g 18%
- Protein: 18.7 g 37%

- Cholesterol: 21 mg 7%
- Sodium: 145 mg 6%

Apple and Kale Smoothie

Ingredients
- 1 cup Nordica 1% or Fat Free Cottage Cheese
- 1 cup unsweetened applesauce
- 1 cup chopped frozen kale or spinach
- 1 small ripe banana
- 1/2 cup water
- 1/2 cup crushed ice
- 1 tablespoon lemon juice
- 1 teaspoon vanilla extract (optional)
- 1/2 teaspoon ground cinnamon
- Add all ingredients to list

Directions
1. Combine cottage cheese, applesauce, kale, banana, water, ice, lemon juice, vanilla (if using) and cinnamon in a blender. Blend on high speed for 2 minutes or until very smooth. Serve immediately.

Nutritional Information
- Calories: 113 kcal 6%
- Fat: 1 g 2%
- Carbs: 18.4g 6%
- Protein: 8.8 g 18%
- Cholesterol: 5 mg 2%
- Sodium: 153 mg 6%

Banana Avocado and Spinach Smoothie

"Quick and delicious smoothie that can be used as a breakfast or snack!"
Serving: *10 m* | **Total Time:** *10 m*

Ingredients
- 1 banana, sliced
- 1/2 avocado, peeled and sliced

- 1/2 cup fresh spinach
- 1/2 cup 1% milk
- 6 ice cubes
- 2 teaspoons honey
- 1 teaspoon vanilla extract
- Add all ingredients to list

Directions

1. Blend banana, avocado, spinach, milk, ice cubes, honey, and vanilla extract together in a blender until smooth.

Nutritional Information

- Calories: 190 kcal 9%
- Fat: 8.2 g 13%
- Carbs: 27.5g 9%
- Protein: 4 g 8%
- Cholesterol: 2 mg < 1%
- Sodium: 45 mg 2%

Banana Mocha Protein Shake

"A delicious, creamy blend of coffee and banana with a hint of chocolate! It's my new favorite way to drink my morning coffee. You'll think you're drinking a milkshake!"
Serving: *5 m |* **Total Time:** *5 m*

Ingredients

- 1 chopped frozen banana
- 1/2 cup chilled brewed coffee
- 1/2 cup unsweetened vanilla-flavored almond milk
- 1/2 cup fresh spinach (optional)
- 1 scoop vanilla protein powder
- 1/2 teaspoon unsweetened cocoa powder
- 1 packet stevia sweetener, or more to taste (optional)
- Add all ingredients to list

Directions

1. Place banana in a blender. Add coffee, almond milk, spinach, protein powder, cocoa powder, and stevia sweetener; blend until smooth.

Nutritional Information
- Calories: 336 kcal 17%
- Fat: 3.2 g 5%
- Carbs: 41.3g 13%
- Protein: 40.1 g 80%
- Cholesterol: 12 mg 4%
- Sodium: 309 mg 12%

Banana Pineapple Green Blend

"Nice quick green smoothie, fairly filling, makes a good snack! Feel free to substitute other fruits, greens, and liquids here! You can add nutmeg, ginger, cloves, cinnamon, and allspice to taste."
Serving: *10 m* | **Total Time:** *10 m*

Ingredients
- 1 cup vanilla soy milk
- 1/2 cup baby spinach leaves
- 1/2 cup water
- 1/2 cup sliced frozen banana
- 1/2 cup chopped frozen pineapple
- Add all ingredients to list

Directions
1. Blend soy milk and spinach together in a blender until spinach is pureed. Add water, banana, and pineapple; blend until smooth.

Nutritional Information
- Calories: 224 kcal 11%
- Fat: 4.1 g 6%
- Carbs: 40.7g 13%
- Protein: 8.2 g 16%
- Cholesterol: 0 mg 0%
- Sodium: 125 mg 5%

Best Green Juice Recipe

"I was experimenting with green juice recipes and finally made a batch I consider to be worth sharing! These ingredients blend together so well that you won't be able to tell there were greens in this drink! I love to have this for breakfast to kick start my day!"
Serving: 10 m | Total Time: 10 m

Ingredients
- 1 Gala apple - peeled, cored, and chopped
- 4 leaves kale, chopped
- 1 cup fresh coconut meat
- 1/2 cucumber, chopped
- 1 stalk celery, chopped
- 1/2 cup spinach
- 1 cup coconut water
- 1/2 cup almond milk
- 1/2 cup water
- 1 lemon, juiced
- Add all ingredients to list

Directions
1. Place apple, kale, coconut meat, cucumber, celery, and spinach in a blender; top with coconut water, almond milk, water, and lemon juice. Blend on high for 30 seconds to 1 minute.

Nutritional Information
- Calories: 126 kcal 6%
- Fat: 7.4 g 11%
- Carbs: 14.8g 5%
- Protein: 2.4 g 5%
- Cholesterol: 0 mg 0%
- Sodium: 108 mg 4%

Blueberry Spinach Protein Smoothie

Ingredients
- 1/2 pint fresh blueberries
- 2 cups fresh spinach
- 1 scoop chocolate-flavored protein powder

- Add all ingredients to list

Directions

1. Combine blueberries, spinach, and protein powder in a blender; blend until smooth.

Nutritional Information
- Calories: 183 kcal 9%
- Fat: 1.8 g 3%
- Carbs: 29.6g 10%
- Protein: 15.9 g 32%
- Cholesterol: 40 mg 13%
- Sodium: 134 mg 5%

Cinnamon Apple Healthy Smoothie

"This is a healthy smoothie drink that has raw spinach in it, but the taste is masked by apples and cinnamon. Tastes wonderful! Add water to mixture if you prefer thinner smoothie drinks."
Serving: *10 m* | **Total Time:** *10 m*

Ingredients
- 1 cup apple juice
- 1 pear, cored and sliced
- 1 apple, cored and sliced
- 1 cup fresh spinach
- 1 teaspoon ground cinnamon
- 1/2 cup ice
- Add all ingredients to list

Directions

1. Pour apple juice into a blender; top with pear, apple, spinach, cinnamon, and ice in that order. Cover and blend until smooth.

Nutritional Information
- Calories: 149 kcal 7%
- Fat: 0.4 g < 1%
- Carbs: 38.3g 12%
- Protein: 1 g 2%

- Cholesterol: 0 mg 0%
- Sodium: 19 mg < 1%

Cool Kale Smoothie

"This is an easy way to get raw kale into your diet. The grapes masks the taste of kale and the end result is a tasty, cool smoothie!"
Serving: *10 m |* **Total Time:** *10 m*

Ingredients
- 2 cups green grapes
- 2 cups kale
- 1 cup ice cubes
- Add all ingredients to list

Directions
1. Blend grapes, kale, and ice together in a blender until smooth.

Nutritional Information
- Calories: 147 kcal 7%
- Fat: 1.4 g 2%
- Carbs: 35.1g 11%
- Protein: 3.3 g 7%
- Cholesterol: 0 mg 0%
- Sodium: 36 mg 1%

Creamy Green Drink

Ingredients
- 2 cups cold water
- 1 cup baby spinach
- 1/2 cup fresh parsley
- 1/2 avocado, peeled and pitted
- 1 tablespoon lemon juice
- 1 teaspoon safflower oil
- Add all ingredients to list

Directions
1. Blend water, spinach, parsley, avocado, lemon juice, and safflower oil together in a blender until smooth.

Nutritional Information
*   Calories: 222 kcal 11%
*   Fat: 19.6 g 30%
*   Carbs: 12.9g 4%
*   Protein: 3.8 g 8%
*   Cholesterol: 0 mg 0%
*   Sodium: 62 mg 2%

Daily Shake

Ingredients
*   1/2 cup Greek yogurt
*   1/2 cup almond milk
*   1/4 cup fresh spinach
*   1/4 cup fresh blueberries
*   1 tablespoon grapeseed oil
*   1 tablespoon ground chia seeds
*   1 tablespoon ground flax seed
*   1 tablespoon ground almonds
*   Add all ingredients to list

Directions
1. Blend yogurt, almond milk, spinach, blueberries, grapeseed oil, chia seeds, flax seed, and almonds together in a blender until smooth.

Nutritional Information
*   Calories: 408 kcal 20%
*   Fat: 31.6 g 49%
*   Carbs: 21.1g 7%
*   Protein: 12.3 g 25%
*   Cholesterol: 22 mg 8%
*   Sodium: 155 mg 6%

Delicious Green Juice

"An easy, delicious green juice. You can substitute kale for spinach."
Serving: *5 m |* **Total Time:** *5 m*

Ingredients
- 1 cup coconut milk
- 1 banana
- 1 mango - peeled, seeded, and chopped
- 3/4 cup fresh spinach, or to taste
- Add all ingredients to list

Directions
1. Blend coconut milk, banana, mango, and spinach together in a blender until smooth.

Nutritional Information
- Calories: 690 kcal 34%
- Fat: 49.2 g 76%
- Carbs: 69.3g 22%
- Protein: 7.6 g 15%
- Cholesterol: 0 mg 0%
- Sodium: 52 mg 2%

Endless Energy

"This is a great recipe to wake you up in the morning. The protein, iron, and fiber will keep you alert until lunch time."
Serving: *10 m |* **Total Time:** *10 m*

Ingredients
- 1 cup almond milk
- 1 cup fresh spinach
- 1 kiwi, peeled and chopped
- 1/2 cup chopped pineapple
- 1/2 cup ice
- Add all ingredients to list

Directions

1.   Blend almond milk, kiwi, spinach, pineapple, and ice in a blender until smooth.

Nutritional Information

- Calories: 157 kcal 8%
- Fat: 3.3 g 5%
- Carbs: 31.3g 10%
- Protein: 3.2 g 6%
- Cholesterol: 0 mg 0%
- Sodium: 190 mg 8%

Energy Elixir Smoothie

Ingredients

- 1 cup spring salad greens, or to taste
- 1 cup frozen red grapes
- 1 chopped frozen banana
- 1 cored and chopped frozen pear
- 2 tablespoons walnuts
- water as needed
- Add all ingredients to list

Directions

1.   Layer salad greens, red grapes, banana, pear, and walnuts in a high-powered blender; add enough water to cover. Blend mixture until smooth, adding more water to reach desired consistency.

Nutritional Information

- Calories: 421 kcal 21%
- Fat: 11.3 g 17%
- Carbs: 84.7g 27%
- Protein: 6.1 g 12%
- Cholesterol: 0 mg 0%
- Sodium: 27 mg 1%

Good Morning Green Smoothie

Ingredients
- 2 cups water
- 1 head romaine lettuce, chopped
- 1/2 cucumber, diced
- 1 avocado, peeled and pitted
- 2 stalks celery
- 2 ounces baby spinach leaves
- lemon, juiced
- 2 cups ice
- 1 apple, cored
- 1 banana
- Add all ingredients to list

Directions
1. Blend water, romaine lettuce, cucumber, avocado, celery, spinach, and lemon juice together in a blender on high until smooth, about 30 seconds. Add ice, apple, and banana to blender and blend until smooth, about 30 seconds.

Nutritional Information
- Calories: 151 kcal 8%
- Fat: 7.9 g 12%
- Carbs: 22.7g 7%
- Protein: 3.3 g 7%
- Cholesterol: 0 mg 0%
- Sodium: 46 mg 2%

Good To Go Morning Smoothie

"I don't usually leave me enough time for breakfast in the morning and came up with this as a quick, healthy smoothie I can put in a to-go cup and drink at work."
Serving: *10 m |* **Total Time:** *10 m*

Ingredients
- 2 cups fresh spinach
- 1 cup rolled oats
- 1 cup apple juice
- 1 banana, sliced

- 2 tablespoons peanut butter
- Add all ingredients to list

Directions
1. Blend spinach, oats, apple juice, banana, and peanut butter together in a blender or food processor until smooth.

Nutritional Information
- Calories: 367 kcal 18%
- Fat: 11.3 g 17%
- Carbs: 59.6g 19%
- Protein: 11 g 22%
- Cholesterol: 0 mg 0%
- Sodium: 105 mg 4%

Grapefruit Smoothie

"A healthy, easy, and satisfying smoothie for those who enjoy grapefruit or are looking for a drink that is lower in sugar and calories. This is loaded with taste and is good for you!"
Serving: *10 m* | ***Total Time:*** *10 m*

Ingredients
- 3 grapefruit, peeled and sectioned
- 1 cup cold water
- 3 ounces fresh spinach
- 6 ice cubes
- 1 (1/2 inch) piece peeled fresh ginger
- 1 teaspoon flax seeds
- Add all ingredients to list

Directions
1. Blend grapefruit, water, spinach, ice cubes, ginger, and flax seeds in a blender or NutriBullet(R) until smooth.

Nutritional Information
- Calories: 201 kcal 10%
- Fat: 1 g 2%
- Carbs: 47.4g 15%

- Protein: 4.6 g 9%
- Cholesterol: 0 mg 0%
- Sodium: 39 mg 2%

Green Banana and Peanut Butter Smoothie

"I saw a Vitamix® demo the other day. Then I realized my Waring Pro® blender at home was already fully capable of the same smoothie greatness, so I got inspired to cram more nutrients into my life by blending them up. The resulting mixture is happy and bright green, but it tastes more like bananas and peanut butter. I can't taste the spinach (though I love it). If it's too thick, use more milk or/and less yogurt and peanut butter. Feel free to substitute nuts for your favorites."
Serving: *10 m |* **Total Time:** *10 m*

Ingredients
- 1/2 cup oats
- 2 tablespoons almonds, or to taste
- 1 cup fresh spinach
- 1 ripe banana
- 2 tablespoons plain yogurt
- 1 tablespoon peanut butter
- 1/8 teaspoon ground cinnamon, or more to taste
- 1 cup rice milk, or as needed
- Add all ingredients to list

Directions
1. Blend oats and almonds in a blender until powdery; add spinach, banana, yogurt, peanut butter, and cinnamon. Blend, gradually adding rice milk, until desired consistency is reached.

Nutritional Information
- Calories: 594 kcal 30%
- Fat: 20 g 31%
- Carbs: 91.4g 29%
- Protein: 18.9 g 38%
- Cholesterol: 2 mg < 1%
- Sodium: 209 mg 8%

Green Breakfast Smoothie

Ingredients
- 2 cups chopped kale
- 1 cup soy milk
- 1 cup fresh spinach
- 1 banana, broken into chunks
- 1/4 cup frozen raspberries
- 1/4 cup frozen pineapple chunks
- Add all ingredients to list

Directions
1. Blend kale, soy milk, spinach, banana, raspberries, and pineapple together in a blender until smooth.

Nutritional Information
- Calories: 377 kcal 19%
- Fat: 5.8 g 9%
- Carbs: 73.3g 24%
- Protein: 15.2 g 30%
- Cholesterol: 0 mg 0%
- Sodium: 208 mg 8%

Green Detox Smoothie

Ingredients
- 3/4 cup pineapple juice
- 1/2 cup fresh spinach leaves
- 1/4 pear, chopped
- 1/4 green apple, chopped
- 1/4 avocado, chopped
- 3 broccoli florets
- Add all ingredients to list

Directions
1. Blend pineapple juice, spinach, pear, apple, avocado, and broccoli florets together in a blender until smooth.

Nutritional Information
- Calories: 379 kcal 19%
- Fat: 9.4 g 15%
- Carbs: 70.2g 23%
- Protein: 15.1 g 30%
- Cholesterol: 0 mg 0%
- Sodium: 169 mg 7%

Green Drink with Aloe Vera Juice

"This is a quick replacement meal!"
Serving: *10 m |* ***Total Time:*** *10 m*

Ingredients
- 1 cup aloe vera juice
- 1/2 cup old-fashioned rolled oats
- 1 cup baby spinach
- 1 cup baby kale
- 1 cup baby chard
- 1 banana
- 1/2 cucumber
- 1/2 cup fresh blueberries
- 2 tablespoons protein powder (optional)
- 1 teaspoon ground cinnamon
- 1 pinch cayenne pepper
- Add all ingredients to list

Directions
1. Mix aloe vera juice and oats together in a bowl; set aside until oats have absorbed the liquid, about 10 minutes.
2. Blend oat mixture, spinach, kale, chard, banana, cucumber, blueberries, protein powder, cinnamon, and cayenne pepper together in a blender until smooth, about 2 minutes.

Nutritional Information
- Calories: 537 kcal 27%
- Fat: 5.2 g 8%
- Carbs: 107.2g 35%
- Protein: 24.3 g 49%
- Cholesterol: 0 mg 0%

- Sodium: 327 mg 13%

Green Monster Smoothie

"Great post-workout snack that will keep you filled for hours! The taste of the banana and the peanut butter cover the taste of the spinach completely. I freeze my bananas and spinach then prepackage everything for the week! Substitutions include rice or nut milks or vanilla yogurt."
Serving: *5 m* | **Total Time:** *5 m*

Ingredients
- 1 cup fat-free milk
- 1/2 cup fat-free plain yogurt
- 1 banana, frozen and chunked
- 1 tablespoon natural peanut butter
- 2 cups fresh spinach
- 1 cup ice cubes (optional)
- Add all ingredients to list

Directions
1. Blend milk, yogurt, banana, peanut butter, spinach, and ice cubes until smooth.

Nutritional Information
- Calories: 382 kcal 19%
- Fat: 9.4 g 14%
- Carbs: 55.7g 18%
- Protein: 23.6 g 47%
- Cholesterol: 7 mg 2%
- Sodium: 335 mg 13%

Green Monster Spinach Smoothie

Ingredients
- 1 cup yogurt
- 1 banana, broken into chunks
- 1/2 cup frozen blueberries
- 4 cups fresh spinach
- 1 tablespoon water, or as desired (optional)

- 2 ice cubes, or as desired (optional)
- Add all ingredients to list

Directions

1. Layer yogurt, banana, and blueberries in a blender, respectively. Add as much spinach to blender that will fit; pour in water. Blend on high speed until smooth, adding the remaining spinach if needed. Add ice for a colder and thicker smoothie. Add more water for a thinner smoothie.

Nutritional Information

- Calories: 164 kcal 8%
- Fat: 2.4 g 4%
- Carbs: 29.5g 10%
- Protein: 9.1 g 18%
- Cholesterol: 7 mg 2%
- Sodium: 135 mg 5%

Green Power Mojito Smoothie

"This tart, satisfying, and delicious smoothie disguises healthy greens with a taste similar to a mojito!"
***Serving:** 10 m | **Total Time:** 10 m*

Ingredients

- 3 cups ice cubes, or as desired
- 2 cups baby spinach leaves, or to taste
- 1 (7 ounce) can crushed pineapple
- 1/2 cup water, or to taste
- 1 banana, broken into chunks
- 1 orange, peeled and segmented
- 10 fresh mint leaves, or more to taste
- 1 lemon, juiced
- 1 lime, juiced
- Add all ingredients to list

Directions

1. Blend ice, spinach, pineapple, water, banana, orange, mint, lemon juice, and lime juice in a blender until smooth.

Nutritional Information
- Calories: 94 kcal 5%
- Fat: 0.3 g < 1%
- Carbs: 24.2g 8%
- Protein: 1.5 g 3%
- Cholesterol: 0 mg 0%
- Sodium: 19 mg < 1%

Green Slime Smoothie

"This is yummy. With a name like this, your kids will love it."
***Serving:** 5 m | **Total Time:** 5 m*

Ingredients
- 2 cups spinach
- 2 cups frozen strawberries
- 1 banana
- 2 tablespoons honey
- 1/2 cup ice
- Add all ingredients to list

Directions
1. Place the spinach in the freezer until frozen, at least 1 hour.
2. Combine the spinach, strawberries, banana, honey, and ice in a blender. Blend until smooth. Serve immediately.

Nutritional Information
- Calories: 100 kcal 5%
- Fat: 0.3 g < 1%
- Carbs: 26g 8%
- Protein: 1.3 g 3%
- Cholesterol: 0 mg 0%
- Sodium: 16 mg < 1%

Green Smoothie Bowl

Ingredients
- Smoothie:

- 3 cups fresh spinach
- 1 banana
- 1/2 (14 ounce) can coconut milk
- 1/2 cup frozen mango chunks
- 1/2 cup coconut water
- Toppings:
- 1/3 cup fresh raspberries
- 1/4 cup fresh blueberries
- 2 tablespoons granola
- 1 tablespoon coconut flakes
- 1/4 teaspoon sliced almonds
- 1/4 teaspoon chia seeds (optional)
- Add all ingredients to list

Directions

1. Blend spinach, banana, coconut milk, mango, and coconut water in a blender until smooth. Pour smoothie into a bowl and top with raspberries, blueberries, granola, coconut flakes, almonds, and chia seeds.

Nutritional Information

- Calories: 374 kcal 19%
- Fat: 25.6 g 39%
- Carbs: 37g 12%
- Protein: 6.3 g 13%
- Cholesterol: 0 mg 0%
- Sodium: 116 mg 5%

Green Smoothie by Karen

Ingredients

- 3 cups water
- 2 cups packed baby kale
- 2 bananas
- 2 1/4 cups apples, seeded
- 2 3/4 cups strawberries
- 1 1/2 cups frozen blackberries
- Add all ingredients to list

Directions

1. Place water, baby kale, bananas, apples, strawberries, and blackberries, respectively, into a heavy-duty blender. Process on high until completely blended.

Nutritional Information

- Calories: 174 kcal 9%
- Fat: 1.1 g 2%
- Carbs: 43g 14%
- Protein: 3.3 g 7%
- Cholesterol: 0 mg 0%
- Sodium: 23 mg < 1%

Green Smoothie with Maca Powder

"Spinach, avocado, banana, almond butter, and maca powder come together in this energizing green smoothie. Carpe diem!"
Serving: *10 m* | **Total Time:** *10 m*

Ingredients

- 2 cups chopped frozen pineapple
- 1 cup fresh spinach
- 1 frozen chopped banana
- 1/2 avocado
- 2 tablespoons almond butter
- 1 teaspoon maca powder
- 3 cups water
- Add all ingredients to list

Directions

1. Layer pineapple, banana, spinach, avocado, almond butter, and maca powder in a blender; pour in water. Blend until smooth.

Nutritional Information

- Calories: 330 kcal 17%
- Fat: 17.3 g 27%
- Carbs: 45.3g 15%
- Protein: 5.9 g 12%
- Cholesterol: 0 mg 0%
- Sodium: 100 mg 4%

Hala Kahiki Green Smoothie

"Hala kahiki is the Hawaiian word for pineapple. This is a seven-ingredient smoothie that is rich in vitamin C and other nutrients. Spinach gives it a beautiful green color yet it tastes tropically sweet. Great for breakfast or a mid-afternoon pick-me-up. Can adjust ice or water to achieve desired thickness of smoothie. I prefer mine not very thick."
Serving: *10 m* | **Total Time:** *10 m*

Ingredients
- 2 oranges, peeled
- 2 cups fresh spinach
- 1 cup water
- 1 cup chopped fresh pineapple
- 1 cup red seedless grapes
- 1 cup crushed ice
- 2 tablespoons ground flax seed (optional)
- Add all ingredients to list

Directions
1. Blend oranges, spinach, water, pineapple, grapes, ice, and flax seed in a blender until smooth.

Nutritional Information
- Calories: 142 kcal 7%
- Fat: 3.6 g 6%
- Carbs: 28.2g 9%
- Protein: 3.1 g 6%
- Cholesterol: 0 mg 0%
- Sodium: 35 mg 1%

Healthy Berry and Spinach Smoothie

"This is an easy way to get kids to eat their veggies. If you want a more fruity taste, exclude the yogurt."
Serving: *10 m* | **Total Time:** *10 m*

Ingredients
- 2 cups frozen berries
- 1 cup plain yogurt
- 1/2 cup orange juice
- 1/4 cup fresh spinach, or to taste
- 5 strawberries
- Add all ingredients to list

Directions
1. Blend berries, yogurt, orange juice, spinach, and strawberries together in a blender until smooth.

Nutritional Information
- Calories: 88 kcal 4%
- Fat: 1.3 g 2%
- Carbs: 17.3g 6%
- Protein: 4.1 g 8%
- Cholesterol: 4 mg 1%
- Sodium: 45 mg 2%

Healthy Caesar Smoothie

Ingredients
- 2 cups tomato and clam juice cocktail (such as Clamato®)
- 1 cup loosely packed fresh spinach
- lemon, juiced
- 1 pinch ground black pepper
- Add all ingredients to list

Directions
1. Blend tomato cocktail, spinach, lemon juice, and ground black pepper together in a blender until smooth.

Nutritional Information
- Calories: 124 kcal 6%
- Fat: 0.1 g < 1%
- Carbs: 28.4g 9%
- Protein: 2 g 4%
- Cholesterol: 0 mg 0%

- Sodium: 892 mg 36%

Healthy Fruit and Vegetable Smoothie

Ingredients
- 6 fluid ounces milk
- 1 (6 ounce) container plain yogurt
- 1/2 cup frozen strawberries
- 1/2 frozen banana
- 1/4 cup frozen blueberries
- 1 green ice cube (see footnote)
- 2 tablespoons whey protein powder (optional)
- 1 teaspoon honey, or to taste
- Add all ingredients to list

Directions
1. Combine milk, yogurt, strawberries, banana, blueberries, green ice cube, whey, and honey in a blender, in the order listed. Blend until smooth.

Nutritional Information
- Calories: 372 kcal 19%
- Fat: 6.8 g 10%
- Carbs: 63.2g 20%
- Protein: 18.1 g 36%
- Cholesterol: 26 mg 9%
- Sodium: 358 mg 14%

Hunter Wellness Mojo Juice

Ingredients
- 1 cup water, divided, or as needed
- 1/2 cup ice, divided, or as needed
- 1 (1/2 inch) piece fresh ginger, peeled
- 2 teaspoons ground cinnamon
- 2 stalks celery
- 1 apple, chopped
- 1/2 cucumber, roughly chopped
- 4 leaves kale

- 1/2 cup fresh spinach, or to taste
- 1/4 cup mixed salad greens, or to taste
- 6 fresh mint leaves, or more to taste
- Add all ingredients to list

Directions

1. Pour 2 fluid ounces water and drop 3 ice cubes into a blender; add ginger and cinnamon. Layer celery, apple, cucumber, kale, spinach, mixed greens, and mint leaves, respectively, in blender. Blend mixture until smooth. Add more water and ice to reach desired consistency.

Nutritional Information

- Calories: 165 kcal 8%
- Fat: 1.3 g 2%
- Carbs: 39.7g 13%
- Protein: 5.4 g 11%
- Cholesterol: 0 mg 0%
- Sodium: 130 mg 5%

Jalapeno Green Smoothie

"Spice up your morning by adding jalapeno pepper to your green smoothie for a refreshing on-the-go breakfast."
Serving: *5 m |* **Total Time:** *5 m*

Ingredients

- 2 bananas, broken into chunks
- 2 cups baby spinach
- 1 cup frozen mango chunks
- 1/2 teaspoon chopped jalapeno pepper, or to taste
- 1 cup water, or as desired
- Add all ingredients to list

Directions

1. Layer banana, spinach, mango, and jalapeno pepper in a blender; add water and blend until smooth, adding more water for a thinner smoothie.

Nutritional Information

- Calories: 166 kcal 8%

- Fat: 0.7 g 1%
- Carbs: 42.1g 14%
- Protein: 2.6 g 5%
- Cholesterol: 0 mg 0%
- Sodium: 30 mg 1%

Jumping Ginger Smoothie

"An amazing smoothie to perk up your morning in place of coffee. Particularly good for a little 'morning after' help. Best with a high-power blender/juicer. I'm a foodie, but not a health-foodie. First and foremost, this thing is crazy delicious. It also happens to be a good way to get more fresh veggies into your day. Bonus!"
Serving: 15 m | Total Time: 15 m

Ingredients
- 2 cups cold water
- 1 avocado, peeled, and pitted
- 1/2 cup fresh parsley
- 1 apple, cored and seeded
- 1 carrot, cut into chunks
- 1 lemon, peeled
- 1 leaf kale leaf, or more to taste
- 1 (1 inch) piece fresh ginger root, or more to taste
- 2 ice cubes (optional)
- 1 tablespoon flax seeds (optional)
- Add all ingredients to list

Directions
1. Blend water, avocado, parsley, apple, carrot, lemon, kale, ginger, ice cubes, and flax seeds in a blender on high until smooth, 10 to 15 seconds.

Nutritional Information
- Calories: 530 kcal 27%
- Fat: 35.7 g 55%
- Carbs: 62.4g 20%
- Protein: 10.1 g 20%
- Cholesterol: 0 mg 0%
- Sodium: 106 mg 4%

Kale and Banana Smoothie

"Nutrient-rich kale is hidden in this delicious banana smoothie. . . perfect for those of us who have a hard time getting our daily dose of veggies!"
Serving: *5 m |* **Total Time:** *5 m*

Ingredients
- 1 banana
- 2 cups chopped kale
- 1/2 cup light unsweetened soy milk
- 1 tablespoon flax seeds
- 1 teaspoon maple syrup
- Add all ingredients to list

Directions
1. Place the banana, kale, soy milk, flax seeds, and maple syrup into a blender. Cover, and puree until smooth. Serve over ice.

Nutritional Information
- Calories: 311 kcal 16%
- Fat: 7.3 g 11%
- Carbs: 56.6g 18%
- Protein: 12.2 g 24%
- Cholesterol: 0 mg 0%
- Sodium: 110 mg 4%

Kale and Berries Breakfast Smoothie

"I eat this every morning because it's quick, easy, and healthy. The berries provide a bunch of antioxidants, the kale packs in the nutrients, and the almonds give it a nice crunch and added protein!"
Serving: *5 m |* **Total Time:** *5 m*

Ingredients
- 1 banana, broken into chunks
- 1/2 cup mixed frozen berries
- 1/2 cup shredded kale
- 1/2 cup orange juice
- 1/2 cup water

- 2 tablespoons plain yogurt
- 10 almonds (optional)
- Add all ingredients to list

Directions

1. Place banana, berries, kale, orange juice, water, yogurt, and almonds into a blender. Cover and puree until smooth, 20 to 30 seconds.

Nutritional Information

- Calories: 296 kcal 15%
- Fat: 7.7 g 12%
- Carbs: 56.2g 18%
- Protein: 7.9 g 16%
- Cholesterol: 2 mg < 1%
- Sodium: 42 mg 2%

Kale Avocado Smoothie

Ingredients

- 1/2 avocado
- 1/2 cup frozen mango chunks
- 1 leaf kale
- 1/2 banana
- 2 tablespoons drained canned white beans
- 1/2 cup water, or more as needed
- Add all ingredients to list

Directions

1. Layer avocado, mango, kale, banana, white beans, and water in a blender; blend until smooth, adding more water for a thinner smoothie.

Nutritional Information

- Calories: 314 kcal 16%
- Fat: 15.4 g 24%
- Carbs: 45g 15%
- Protein: 6.1 g 12%
- Cholesterol: 0 mg 0%
- Sodium: 23 mg < 1%

Kale Banana and Peanut Butter Smoothie

"My own little concoction for a quick and healthy snack on the go."
Serving: *10 m* | **Total Time:** *10 m*

Ingredients
- 2 bananas, cut into small chunks
- 1 1/2 cups unsweetened vanilla-flavored almond milk
- 1/2 bunch kale - stems removed and discarded, leaves torn into bite-size pieces
- 4 cubes ice, or more if desired
- 1 tablespoon peanut butter
- Add all ingredients to list

Directions
1. Blend bananas, almond milk, kale, ice, and peanut butter in a blender until smooth.

Nutritional Information
- Calories: 563 kcal 28%
- Fat: 14.6 g 22%
- Carbs: 105.3g 34%
- Protein: 15.7 g 31%
- Cholesterol: 0 mg 0%
- Sodium: 417 mg 17%

Kale Banana Smoothie

"So good! Great flavor and not too sweet. Very filling!"
Serving: *10 m* | **Total Time:** *10 m*

Ingredients
- 16 fluid ounces coconut water, chilled
- 1 banana
- 1/2 avocado, peeled and pitted
- 1/2 cup packed kale
- 1/8 lemon, juiced
- 1 pinch cayenne pepper

- Add all ingredients to list

Directions
1. Put coconut water, banana, avocado, kale, lemon juice, and cayenne pepper in blender; blend until smooth, about 30 seconds.

Nutritional Information
- Calories: 371 kcal 19%
- Fat: 16.3 g 25%
- Carbs: 56.2g 18%
- Protein: 7.8 g 16%
- Cholesterol: 0 mg 0%
- Sodium: 510 mg 20%

Kale Orange Banana Smoothie

"Sometimes it tastes like Fruit Loops® cereal, but, of course, this is actually good for you. My 14-month-old loves this for breakfast. Furthermore, he can feed himself (with a sippy cup) while I make breakfast and lunch for the older kids. The texture is similar to pudding. If runnier texture is desired, add ice or milk."
***Serving:** 10 m | **Total Time:** 10 m*

Ingredients
- 1 orange, peeled
- 1/2 cup water
- 1 leaf kale, torn into several pieces
- 2 ripe bananas, peeled
- Add all ingredients to list

Directions
1. Blend the orange in a blender until mostly juice.
2. Add the water and kale; blend again on High speed until kale is liquefied.
3. Break the bananas into chunks and add to the blender. Start blending on a lower speed until the banana is incorporated. Increase speed to blend the mixture into a pudding-like texture.

Nutritional Information
- Calories: 220 kcal 11%
- Fat: 0.9 g 1%
- Carbs: 55.9g 18%

- Protein: 3.2 g 6%
- Cholesterol: 0 mg 0%
- Sodium: 15 mg < 1%

Kale Smoothie

Ingredients
- 1 cup chopped kale
- 1 cup chopped fresh spinach
- 1 cup pineapple juice
- 1 cup orange juice
- 1 1/2 cups chopped fresh pineapple
- 1 small yellow mango - peeled, pitted, and roughly chopped
- Add all ingredients to list

Directions
1. Place kale and spinach in a blender; blend until leaves become finely chopped. Add pineapple juice and orange juice; blend until smooth. Add pineapple and mango; blend until smooth.

Nutritional Information
- Calories: 157 kcal 8%
- Fat: 0.5 g < 1%
- Carbs: 39g 13%
- Protein: 1.9 g 4%
- Cholesterol: 0 mg 0%
- Sodium: 12 mg < 1%

Kalenutsco

Ingredients
- 2 cups coconut water
- 4 leaves kale
- 1 cup walnuts
- 1/2 cup shredded sweetened coconut
- Add all ingredients to list

Directions

1. Blend coconut water, kale, walnuts, and coconut in a blender until smooth; refrigerate up to 1 hour.

Nutritional Information

* Calories: 181 kcal 9%
* Fat: 15 g 23%
* Carbs: 10.2g 3%
* Protein: 4.3 g 9%
* Cholesterol: 0 mg 0%
* Sodium: 108 mg 4%

Kiwi Sensation

"This is a green smoothie that I created for the September challenge of BlackWomenLosingWeight.com. Makes about 16 ounces! Prep time depends on whether the mango and kiwi are already peeled and sliced."
Serving: *10 m* | **Total Time:** *10 m*

Ingredients

* 1 kiwi, peeled and sliced
* 1/2 cup pineapple chunks
* 1/2 cup green grapes
* 1/4 mango - peeled, seeded, and diced
* 1/4 cup water
* 1/2 cup spinach
* 2 cubes ice cubes, or as needed
* Add all ingredients to list

Directions

1. Blend kiwi, pineapple, grapes, mango, and water in a blender until smooth. Add spinach and blend again until spinach is completely integrated. Add ice and blend until ice is completely integrated.

Nutritional Information

* Calories: 102 kcal 5%
* Fat: 0.6 g < 1%
* Carbs: 25.8g 8%
* Protein: 1.3 g 3%
* Cholesterol: 0 mg 0%

- Sodium: 10 mg < 1%

Lean and Green

Ingredients
- 1 cup fresh spinach
- 1 banana
- 1/2 green apple
- 4 hulled strawberries
- 4 (1 inch) pieces frozen mango
- 1/3 cup whole milk
- 1 scoop vanilla protein powder (optional)
- 1 teaspoon honey
- Add all ingredients to list

Directions
1. Blend spinach, banana, apple, strawberries, mango, milk, protein powder, and honey together in a blender until smooth.

Nutritional Information
- Calories: 456 kcal 23%
- Fat: 4.9 g 8%
- Carbs: 66.9g 22%
- Protein: 43.3 g 87%
- Cholesterol: 21 mg 7%
- Sodium: 273 mg 11%

Lemon Coconut Cleanser

Ingredients
- 1 cup frozen mango chunks
- 1/2 lemon, peeled
- 1 cup fresh spinach
- 1/4 unpeeled zucchini, chopped
- 3/4 cup water
- 4 ice cubes, or more to taste
- 1 tablespoon coconut oil, melted

- Add all ingredients to list

Directions

1. Combine mango chunks, lemon, spinach, zucchini, water, ice cubes, and coconut oil in a high-speed blender; blend until smooth.

Nutritional Information

- Calories: 79 kcal 4%
- Fat: 7 g 11%
- Carbs: 6.4g 2%
- Protein: 1 g 2%
- Cholesterol: 0 mg 0%
- Sodium: 18 mg < 1%

Lemon Spinach Mint Smoothie

Ingredients

- 1 cup fresh spinach, or more to taste
- 1/2 banana
- 1/2 avocado
- 1 kiwi, peeled and ends removed
- 1 lemon, juiced
- 10 mint leaves
- 6 raw almonds
- 1 tablespoon maple syrup
- 1 teaspoon flax seeds
- 1 cup cold water, or as needed to cover
- 3 ice cubes
- Add all ingredients to list

Directions

1. Combine spinach, banana, avocado, kiwi, lemon juice, mint, almonds, maple syrup, and flax seeds in a blender. Add enough water to almost cover ingredients; blend until smooth. Add ice and blend thoroughly.

Nutritional Information

- Calories: 243 kcal 12%
- Fat: 8.2 g 13%
- Carbs: 42.6g 14%

- Protein: 4.9 g 10%
- Cholesterol: 0 mg 0%
- Sodium: 40 mg 2%

Liquid Green Platinum Drink

Ingredients
- 1 cup chopped fresh kale
- 1 cup baby spinach
- 1 cup fresh parsley
- 1 cup pineapple juice, or more to taste
- 1 fresh pineapple spear (optional)
- Add all ingredients to list

Directions
1. Blend kale, spinach, parsley, pineapple juice, and pineapple in a blender until smooth.

Nutritional Information
- Calories: 222 kcal 11%
- Fat: 1.4 g 2%
- Carbs: 51.1g 16%
- Protein: 6.1 g 12%
- Cholesterol: 0 mg 0%
- Sodium: 92 mg 4%

Mango Pineapple Green Smoothie

"A yummy, healthy smoothie made with mangoes, pineapple, banana, and spinach (shhhh!) that's sure to be a hit!"
***Serving:** 10 m | **Total Time:** 10 m*

Ingredients
- 2/3 cup frozen pineapple chunks
- 1 cup frozen mango chunks
- 1 ripe banana, sliced
- 2/3 cup fresh spinach
- 1/3 cup orange juice

- 1 cup ice
- Add all ingredients to list

Directions
1. Place pineapple, mango, banana, spinach, orange juice, and ice, respectively, in a blender and blend until smooth.

Nutritional Information
- Calories: 197 kcal 10%
- Fat: 0.6 g < 1%
- Carbs: 50.3g 16%
- Protein: 2 g 4%
- Cholesterol: 0 mg 0%
- Sodium: 16 mg < 1%

Matcha Berry Swirl Smoothie

Ingredients
- 2 cups fresh spinach
- 2 cups orange juice, divided
- 1 cup frozen peaches
- 1 cup frozen pineapple chunks
- 2 frozen bananas, halved, divided
- 2 teaspoons green tea powder (matcha)
- 1 cup frozen raspberries
- 1 cup frozen strawberries
- Add all ingredients to list

Directions
1. Combine spinach, 1 cup orange juice, peaches, pineapple, 1 halved banana, and green tea powder in a blender; blend until combined. Pour smoothie into a glass.
2. Rinse out the blender.
3. Combine 1 cup orange juice, raspberries, strawberries, and 1 halved banana in the blender; blend until combined. Pour berry smoothie into a separate glass.
4. Combine smoothies by pouring them at the same time from opposite sides of the serving glass.

Nutritional Information
- Calories: 262 kcal 13%

- Fat: 0.7 g 1%
- Carbs: 65.6g 21%
- Protein: 3.3 g 7%
- Cholesterol: 0 mg 0%
- Sodium: 17 mg < 1%

Matcha Coconut Smoothie

Ingredients
- 1 banana
- 1 cup frozen mango chunks
- 2 leaves kale, torn into several pieces
- 3 tablespoons white beans, drained
- 2 tablespoons unsweetened shredded coconut
- 1/2 teaspoon matcha green tea powder
- 1 cup water
- Add all ingredients to list

Directions
1. Combine banana, mango, kale, white beans, coconut, and matcha powder in a blender; add water. Blend mixture until very smooth.

Nutritional Information
- Calories: 367 kcal 18%
- Fat: 8.8 g 14%
- Carbs: 72.4g 23%
- Protein: 8 g 16%
- Cholesterol: 0 mg 0%
- Sodium: 36 mg 1%

Power Packed Smoothie

Ingredients
- 1 cup cold water
- 1 small banana
- 1/2 cup spinach, or more to taste
- 1 teaspoon spirulina powder

- Add all ingredients to list

Directions

1. Place cold water, banana, and spinach leaves in a blender; blend to combine, about 5 seconds. Add spirulina powder and blend until smooth, 1 minute more.

Nutritional Information

- Calories: 100 kcal 5%
- Fat: 0.6 g < 1%
- Carbs: 24.2g 8%
- Protein: 2.9 g 6%
- Cholesterol: 0 mg 0%
- Sodium: 44 mg 2%

Protein Packed Spinach Smoothie

Ingredients

- 2 cups fresh spinach leaves
- 2 bananas, cut into chunks
- 1 ounce firm tofu
- 2 tablespoons unsweetened shredded coconut
- 1/2 cup frozen peach slices
- 1/2 cup frozen pineapple chunks
- 1/2 cup frozen mango chunks
- 1/2 cup frozen strawberries
- 1 cup unsweetened apple juice, or to taste
- Add all ingredients to list

Directions

1. Place spinach, bananas, tofu, coconut, peaches, pineapple, mango, and strawberries, respectively, in a blender; pour in apple juice. Blend until desired consistency is reached, adding more apple juice as necessary.

Nutritional Information

- Calories: 377 kcal 19%
- Fat: 5.4 g 8%
- Carbs: 84.8g 27%
- Protein: 4.8 g 10%
- Cholesterol: 0 mg 0%

- Sodium: 39 mg 2%

Quick Green Smoothie

"A quick, healthy breakfast for anyone on the go. Substitute any liquid for the milk."
Serving: *10 m* | **Total Time:** *10 m*

Ingredients
- 1 cup stemmed kale
- 1 cup skim milk
- 1 sliced frozen banana
- 1/2 green apple, cut into chunks
- 1/2 pear, cut into chunks
- 1/4 cup old-fashioned rolled oats
- 1 tablespoon peanut butter
- 1 tablespoon flax seed meal
- 1 tablespoon wheat germ
- 2 sprigs fresh parsley, or more to taste
- Add all ingredients to list

Directions
1. Blend kale, milk, banana, apple, pear, oats, peanut butter, flax seed meal, wheat germ, and parsley in a blender until smooth.

Nutritional Information
- Calories: 561 kcal 28%
- Fat: 14.9 g 23%
- Carbs: 94.3g 30%
- Protein: 23.6 g 47%
- Cholesterol: 5 mg 2%
- Sodium: 245 mg 10%

Quick Kale and Banana Smoothie

"Very easy and fruity and the kids loved it. Using the coconut milk, banana, and frozen strawberries cut down on any bitterness from the kale."
Serving: *10 m* | **Total Time:** *10 m*

Ingredients
- 2 cups chopped kale
- 1 banana, cut into chunks
- 1/2 cup coconut milk
- 1/2 cup frozen strawberries, or more to taste
- Add all ingredients to list

Directions
1. Blend kale, banana, coconut milk, and strawberries together in a blender until smooth.

Nutritional Information
- Calories: 433 kcal 22%
- Fat: 25.6 g 39%
- Carbs: 53.6g 17%
- Protein: 8.5 g 17%
- Cholesterol: 0 mg 0%
- Sodium: 76 mg 3%

Quick Kale and Turmeric Smoothie

"This is a quick meal replacement, detox vitamin-packed drink. You will love it!"
***Serving:** 5 m | **Total Time:** 5 m*

Ingredients
- 6 ice cubes
- 1 cup almond milk
- 1 banana
- 3 leaves kale, large stems discarded, leaves chopped
- 1/4 cup flax seed meal
- 2 tablespoons chopped fresh ginger
- 2 tablespoons chopped fresh turmeric root
- 1 tablespoon almond butter
- 1/4 teaspoon stevia
- 1/4 teaspoon cayenne pepper
- 1/8 teaspoon ground black pepper
- Add all ingredients to list

Directions

1. Blend ice cubes, almond milk, banana, kale, flax seed meal, ginger, turmeric root, almond butter, stevia powder, cayenne pepper, and ground black pepper together in a blender until smooth.

Nutritional Information

- Calories: 471 kcal 24%
- Fat: 25 g 38%
- Carbs: 58.1g 19%
- Protein: 12.4 g 25%
- Cholesterol: 0 mg 0%
- Sodium: 274 mg 11%

Raw Mango Monster Smoothie

"The raw adventure continues this morning with my satisfying Mango Monster Smoothie. Why is it a monster smoothie you ask? It's green, that's why...and green makes me think of monsters. This smoothie is so yummy and you can feel great drinking it because of how good it is for you!"
Serving: 10 m | Total Time: 10 m

Ingredients

- 1 tablespoon flax seeds
- 2 tablespoons pepitas (raw pumpkin seeds)
- 1 ripe mango, cubed
- 1 frozen banana, quartered
- 1/3 cup water, or more to taste
- 3 ice cubes
- 2 leaves kale, or more to taste
- Add all ingredients to list

Directions

1. Blend flax seeds in a blender until finely ground; add pepitas and blend until ground, about 1 minute.
2. Place mango, banana, water, ice cubes, and kale in the blender; blend until smooth, kale is fully incorporated, and the smoothie is uniform in color, about 3 minutes. Thin with more water to reach desired consistency.

Nutritional Information

- Calories: 381 kcal 19%

- Fat: 14.1 g 22%
- Carbs: 63g 20%
- Protein: 9.8 g 20%
- Cholesterol: 0 mg 0%
- Sodium: 32 mg 1%

Salad Smoothie

"Going raw is a great lifestyle choice. You can find a lot of fruit smoothies that taste good. Here is a great vegetable one too."
***Serving:** 10 m | **Total Time:** 10 m*

Ingredients
- 1 cup water, or as desired
- 1/2 orange, peeled
- 1 cup fresh spinach
- 1/2 raw beet, peeled
- 1/3 cup baby carrots
- 1/3 cup cauliflower florets
- 1/3 cup broccoli florets
- 1/4 cup blueberries, or to taste
- 1 stalk celery
- 1/2 lime, peeled
- 1 tablespoon honey
- 1 tablespoon chia seeds
- Add all ingredients to list

Directions
1. Pour water into the pitcher of a high-powered blender; add the orange, spinach, beet, carrots, cauliflower, broccoli, blueberries, celery, lime, honey, and chia seeds. Blend on high speed until smooth, about 1 minute.

Nutritional Information
- Calories: 199 kcal 10%
- Fat: 3 g 5%
- Carbs: 43.6g 14%
- Protein: 5.5 g 11%
- Cholesterol: 0 mg 0%
- Sodium: 149 mg 6%

Secret Ingredient Smoothie

Ingredients
- 3 cups chopped romaine lettuce
- 1/3 cup milk, or more as needed
- 4 frozen strawberries, or more to taste
- 1 frozen banana, cut into chunks
- 1/4 teaspoon vanilla extract, or to taste (optional)
- Add all ingredients to list

Directions
1. Put romaine lettuce into the bottom of a blender pitcher; add enough milk to cover completely and blend on High until smooth.
2. Drop one strawberry at a time into the blender while still running on High and allow the berry to blend completely before adding the next. Blend one banana chunk at a time into the mixture in the same manner as the strawberries. Thin the smoothie with additional milk to keep smoothie blending properly. Blend vanilla extract into the smoothie.

Nutritional Information
- Calories: 200 kcal 10%
- Fat: 2.7 g 4%
- Carbs: 42g 14%
- Protein: 6.5 g 13%
- Cholesterol: 7 mg 2%
- Sodium: 49 mg 2%

Sesame Mango Smoothie

Ingredients
- 1 banana
- 1 cup frozen mango chunks
- 1 small cucumber, roughly chopped
- 2 cups fresh spinach
- 2 tablespoons cashew butter
- 1 teaspoon toasted sesame seeds
- 1 cup water
- Add all ingredients to list

Directions

1. Layer banana, mango, cucumber, spinach, cashew butter, and sesame seeds in a blender, in the order mentioned; add water. Blend until smoothie is desired consistency, adding more water if desired.

Nutritional Information

- Calories: 183 kcal 9%
- Fat: 9.1 g 14%
- Carbs: 24.6g 8%
- Protein: 5.2 g 10%
- Cholesterol: 0 mg 0%
- Sodium: 128 mg 5%

Skinny Black Forest Smoothie

"A thick and creamy skinny Black Forest smoothie made with blended chocolate, cherry, milk, and spinach. A delicious smoothie packed with antioxidants and fiber. The perfect post-workout smoothie that doubles as a dessert!"
Serving: *10 m |* **Total Time:** *10 m*

Ingredients

- 2 cups baby spinach
- 1 cup frozen cherries
- 1 cup almond milk
- 1/4 cup rolled oats
- 2 tablespoons unsweetened cocoa powder
- 1 packet stevia sweetener (such as Truvia®)
- 1 teaspoon chia seeds, or to taste (optional)
- Add all ingredients to list

Directions

1. Place baby spinach, cherries, almond milk, rolled oats, cocoa powder, and sweetener in a blender. Blend until smooth, about 2 minutes. Pour into a glass and top with chia seeds.

Nutritional Information

- Calories: 264 kcal 13%
- Fat: 7.1 g 11%
- Carbs: 49.4g 16%
- Protein: 9.4 g 19%

- Cholesterol: 0 mg 0%
- Sodium: 213 mg 9%

Spinach and Banana Power Smoothie

"A quick, easy and surprisingly delicious vegan pick-me-up that makes the most of raw superfoods and protein-rich soy. I make one of these healthy treats for myself every morning for breakfast, and it powers me all the way until lunch. I love the mild sweetness of the banana, but if you want it sweeter you could add sugar. I've also added different things like fresh ginger, cinnamon, apple, or any number of other things. Raw vegans can substitute raw almond milk for the soy. Feel free to experiment with different flavors, and enjoy the pure energy that comes from eating delicious and good-for-you food!"
*Serving: 10 m | **Total Time:** 10 m*

Ingredients
- 1 cup plain soy milk
- 3/4 cup packed fresh spinach leaves
- 1 large banana, sliced
- Add all ingredients to list

Directions
1. Blend soy milk and spinach leaves together in a blender until smooth. Add banana and pulse until thoroughly blended.

Nutritional Information
- Calories: 257 kcal 13%
- Fat: 4.8 g 7%
- Carbs: 47.1g 15%
- Protein: 10.1 g 20%
- Cholesterol: 0 mg 0%
- Sodium: 143 mg 6%

Spinach and Berry Smoothie with Truvia® Natural Sweetener

"Also known as the 'Green Dream' this beverage is a refreshing, non-dairy smoothie that contains fresh spinach and has 25% fewer calories and 30% less sugar than the full-sugar version."

*Serving: 10 m | **Total Time:** 10 m*

Ingredients

- 1 cup fresh strawberries
- 1 banana
- 1 cup orange juice
- 1 cup almond milk
- 2 cups fresh baby spinach
- 1 cup ice
- 4 (3.5 gram) packets Truvia® natural sweetener, or more to desired level of sweetness
- Add all ingredients to list

Directions

1. Add all ingredients into a blender.
2. Blend on high until smooth.

Nutritional Information

- Calories: 86 kcal 4%
- Fat: 1.1 g 2%
- Carbs: 21.8g 7%
- Protein: 1.7 g 3%
- Cholesterol: 0 mg 0%
- Sodium: 55 mg 2%

Spinach and Kale Smoothie

"A delicious way to add more veggies to your diet! This recipe is very versatile. You can change out the greens with whatever you want. Chia seeds give you added protein and energy. Hemp seeds will give you a boost of omegas!"
*Serving: 10 m | **Total Time:** 10 m*

Ingredients

- 2 cups fresh spinach
- 1 cup almond milk
- 1 tablespoon peanut butter
- 1 tablespoon chia seeds (optional)
- 1 leaf kale
- 1 sliced frozen banana

- Add all ingredients to list

Directions

1. Blend spinach, almond milk, peanut butter, chia seeds, and kale together in a blender until smooth. Add banana and blend until smooth.

Nutritional Information

- Calories: 325 kcal 16%
- Fat: 13.9 g 21%
- Carbs: 46.1g 15%
- Protein: 10 g 20%
- Cholesterol: 0 mg 0%
- Sodium: 293 mg 12%

Spinach Power

Ingredients

- 1 large cucumber, chopped
- 2 apples, cored and chopped
- 3 ribs celery, chopped
- 1/2 cup cold water, or more as needed
- 2 cups fresh spinach
- 1 bunch fresh parsley
- 1 (1 inch) piece fresh ginger, peeled and chopped
- 1 lime, juiced
- 1/2 lemon, juiced
- Add all ingredients to list

Directions

1. Place cucumber, apples, celery, water, spinach, parsley, ginger, lime juice, and lemon juice in a blender; blend until smooth.

Nutritional Information

- Calories: 89 kcal 4%
- Fat: 0.6 g < 1%
- Carbs: 21.4g 7%
- Protein: 2.5 g 5%
- Cholesterol: 0 mg 0%
- Sodium: 83 mg 3%

Stellar Kale Smoothie

Ingredients
- 1 cup chopped fresh pineapple
- 8 pitted dates
- 1 tablespoon vanilla extract
- 1/4 cup frozen blackberries, or to taste
- 1/2 cup chopped kale leaves
- 1 cup chopped frozen pineapple
- Add all ingredients to list

Directions
1. Blend fresh pineapple, dates, and vanilla extract together in a Vitamix(R) or blender until smooth, about 90 seconds. Add blackberries and blend, about 90 seconds. Add kale and blend, about 90 seconds; repeat for 90 seconds more. Add frozen pineapple and blend until smooth, about 90 seconds.

Nutritional Information
- Calories: 141 kcal 7%
- Fat: 0.4 g < 1%
- Carbs: 33.9g 11%
- Protein: 1.7 g 3%
- Cholesterol: 0 mg 0%
- Sodium: 7 mg < 1%

Super Fresh Smoothie

Ingredients
- 1 banana
- 4 leaves kale
- 1/2 lime, juiced
- 1 tablespoon honey, or more to taste (optional)
- Add all ingredients to list

Directions
1. Combine banana, kale, lime juice, and honey in a blender; blend until smooth.

Nutritional Information
- Calories: 211 kcal 11%
- Fat: 1 g 1%
- Carbs: 52.9g 17%
- Protein: 4 g 8%
- Cholesterol: 0 mg 0%
- Sodium: 37 mg 1%

Super Green Tea Smoothie

Ingredients
- 1 cup brewed green tea (such as Gold Peak®), chilled
- 1 cup fresh spinach leaves
- 1 kiwi, peeled
- 1/4 avocado
- 1 banana, broken into chunks and frozen
- 1/2 teaspoon grated fresh ginger
- Add all ingredients to list

Directions
1. Combine tea, spinach, kiwi, avocado, banana, and ginger in a blender. Blend until smooth.

Nutritional Information
- Calories: 120 kcal 6%
- Fat: 4.1 g 6%
- Carbs: 22g 7%
- Protein: 2 g 4%
- Cholesterol: 0 mg 0%
- Sodium: 19 mg < 1%

Superfood Berry Green Smoothie

"This is a meal-sized breakfast smoothie that will fill you up from morning until lunch. High in anti-oxidants, fiber, protein, and vitamin C, this smoothie is both tasty and healthy!"
*Serving: 10 m | **Total Time:** 10 m*

Ingredients

- 1 1/4 cups unsweetened almond milk
- 1 clementine (such as Cuties®), peeled
- 1/2 cup frozen raspberries
- 1 cup spinach, or more to taste
- 1 tablespoon chia seeds
- 1 tablespoon flaxseed meal
- 1 cup frozen blueberries
- 1 scoop vanilla protein powder
- Add all ingredients to list

Directions

1. Place almond milk, clementine, raspberries, spinach, chia seeds, flaxseed meal, blueberries, and protein powder in the blender, respectively. Blend on high until smooth, about 30 seconds.

Nutritional Information

- Calories: 490 kcal 24%
- Fat: 11.5 g 18%
- Carbs: 58g 19%
- Protein: 44 g 88%
- Cholesterol: 12 mg 4%
- Sodium: 443 mg 18%

Superfood Green Smoothie

Ingredients

- 1 cup spinach leaves
- 1 cup shredded kale
- 1/2 pear, cut into chunks
- 1/2 large ripe banana, sliced
- 1/2 cup frozen blueberries
- 1/3 cup plain yogurt
- 4 ice cubes
- 2 tablespoons ground flax seeds
- 1/2 cup brewed green tea, chilled, or more to taste
- Add all ingredients to list

Directions

1. Combine spinach, kale, pear, banana, blueberries, yogurt, ice cubes, and ground flax seeds in a blender; pour in tea. Blend on high until mixture is smooth. Mix with a wooden spoon to redistribute ingredients if needed.

Nutritional Information

- Calories: 175 kcal 9%
- Fat: 6.3 g 10%
- Carbs: 27.4g 9%
- Protein: 5.9 g 12%
- Cholesterol: 2 mg < 1%
- Sodium: 54 mg 2%

Terri's Spicy Vegetable Smoothie

Ingredients

- 1/2 cup fresh spinach, or more to taste
- 1 carrot, roughly chopped
- 1 rib celery
- 1 small tomato, halved
- 1/2 apple, cored
- 1/2 lime, juiced
- 1 tablespoon ground flaxseed
- 1 (1/2 inch) piece fresh ginger, peeled
- 1 pinch salt-free seasoning blend (such as Mrs. Dash® Southwest Chipotle), or to taste
- 1 dash hot sauce (such as Frank's RedHot ®), or to taste
- 1 dash Worcestershire sauce, or to taste
- water to cover
- Add all ingredients to list

Directions

1. Combine spinach, carrot, celery, tomato, apple, lime juice, ground flaxseed, ginger, seasoning blend, hot sauce, and Worcestershire sauce in a blender; add enough water to cover. Blend mixture until smooth.

Nutritional Information

- Calories: 136 kcal 7%
- Fat: 3.6 g 6%
- Carbs: 25.6g 8%

- Protein: 3.8 g 8%
- Cholesterol: 0 mg 0%
- Sodium: 150 mg 6%

The Drink by Will

"My green savory drink. I couldn't find a recipe that I liked online, so I made my own. I use a Vitamix® 7500 and crank it up to 7 or 8 for 35 to 45 seconds and it's smooth and drinkable. I blend rather than juice because I can't rationalize throwing out fruit/vegetable pulp. Throw one of these back every day and feel the power! Let me know what you think."
Serving: 10 m | Total Time: 10 m

Ingredients
- 1 cup water
- 1 tomato, roughly chopped
- 1 large carrot, roughly chopped
- 1 cup kale
- 2 radishes, roughly chopped
- 1 lemon, peeled
- 1 teaspoon spirulina powder
- 6 ice cubes, or as needed
- Add all ingredients to list

Directions
1. Pour water into a blender. Add tomato, carrot, kale, radishes, lemon, spirulina powder; top with ice cubes. Blend vegetable mixture until smooth.

Nutritional Information
- Calories: 98 kcal 5%
- Fat: 1.1 g 2%
- Carbs: 20.3g 7%
- Protein: 5.6 g 11%
- Cholesterol: 0 mg 0%
- Sodium: 125 mg 5%

Thin Mint Green Monster

"A delicious (though a bit odd looking) smoothie that is dairy free and fills that chocolate-mint craving!"
***Serving:** 10 m | **Total Time:** 10 m*

Ingredients
* 1/2 cup chilled coconut milk
* 1 cup fresh spinach leaves
* 10 leaves fresh mint, chopped
* 1/4 cup raw cacao seeds
* 1 teaspoon peppermint extract
* 1 (1 gram) packet stevia powder
* 1 banana, cut into pieces and frozen
* ice, or as needed
* water, or as needed
* Add all ingredients to list

Directions
1. Blend coconut milk, spinach, mint leaves, cacao seeds, peppermint extract, and stevia powder in a blender. While blender is running, drop in banana chunks, one by one. Add ice cubes until smoothie has desired thickness, and water if smoothie is too thick.

Nutritional Information
* Calories: 173 kcal 9%
* Fat: 12.3 g 19%
* Carbs: 16.2g 5%
* Protein: 2.2 g 4%
* Cholesterol: 0 mg 0%
* Sodium: 21 mg < 1%

Tropical Smoothie with Kale

"Don't be afraid of kale! This tropical smoothie tastes more like pineapple and banana, it just happens to be bright green."
***Serving:** 10 m | **Total Time:** 10 m*

Ingredients
- 1 1/2 cups frozen pineapple chunks
- 1 cup chopped kale
- 1 banana, cut in chunks
- 1 cup almond milk, or as needed
- Add all ingredients to list

Directions
1. Place pineapple, kale, and banana in a NutriBullet(R) or blender; add almond milk. Blend until smooth.

Nutritional Information
- Calories: 163 kcal 8%
- Fat: 1.9 g 3%
- Carbs: 37.3g 12%
- Protein: 2.9 g 6%
- Cholesterol: 0 mg 0%
- Sodium: 96 mg 4%

Vegan Green Smoothie

Ingredients
- 2 cups coconut water
- 1 cup baby spinach
- 1 banana
- 6 sliced fresh strawberries
- 5 dates, pitted
- Add all ingredients to list

Directions
1. Blend coconut water, spinach, banana, strawberries, and dates together in a blender.

Nutritional Information
- Calories: 118 kcal 6%
- Fat: 0.7 g 1%
- Carbs: 28.4g 9%
- Protein: 2.4 g 5%
- Cholesterol: 0 mg 0%

- Sodium: 177 mg 7%

Veggie Fruit and Nut Nutritious Green Smoothie!

Ingredients
- 1 1/2 cups baby spinach leaves
- 1 cup shredded carrots
- 1/2 cup sliced raw beet
- 1/2 pear, cored and chopped
- 1/2 cup milk
- 1/2 banana, sliced
- 1/4 cup cottage cheese
- 1/4 cup walnut halves
- 1/4 cup whole almonds
- 2 tablespoons Greek yogurt
- 1 tablespoon honey
- 1/2 teaspoon ground cinnamon
- Add all ingredients to list

Directions
1. Blend spinach, carrots, beet, pear, milk, banana, cottage cheese, walnuts, almonds, yogurt, honey, and cinnamon together in a blender until smooth.

Nutritional Information
- Calories: 386 kcal 19%
- Fat: 21.3 g 33%
- Carbs: 40.9g 13%
- Protein: 14.2 g 28%
- Cholesterol: 12 mg 4%
- Sodium: 231 mg 9%

Wild Pina Colada Green Smoothie

Ingredients
- 4 cups fresh diced pineapple
- 2 cups coconut water
- 2 cups ice cubes
- 1 cup chopped dandelion greens

- 1/2 cup shredded unsweetened coconut
- 1/4 cup cashews
- 1/4 cup chopped pitted dates, or more to taste
- Add all ingredients to list

Directions

1. Blend pineapple, coconut water, ice cubes, dandelion greens, coconut, cashews, and dates in a blender until smooth and creamy.

Nutritional Information

- Calories: 263 kcal 13%
- Fat: 12 g 19%
- Carbs: 39.8g 13%
- Protein: 4.5 g 9%
- Cholesterol: 0 mg 0%
- Sodium: 201 mg 8%

Winter Refresher Green Smoothie

Ingredients

- 1 cup water
- 1 cup fresh spinach leaves, or to taste
- 1 apple, cored and quartered
- 1 orange, peeled
- 1 cucumber, peeled and quartered
- 1/2 cup cranberries
- 1 (1/2 inch) piece fresh ginger root, peeled
- Add all ingredients to list

Directions

1. Place water, spinach, apple, orange, cucumber, cranberries, and ginger in a blender. Blend on low until just combined; increase speed to high and blend until smooth and liquefied, about 1 minute.

Nutritional Information

- Calories: 33 kcal 2%
- Fat: 0.2 g < 1%
- Carbs: 8.1g 3%
- Protein: 0.7 g 1%

- Cholesterol: 0 mg 0%
- Sodium: 9 mg < 1%

Chapter 6: Mango Smoothies

***

Basic Fruit Smoothie

"This is a great smoothie consisting of fruit, fruit juice and ice. I like to use whatever fresh fruits I crave that day. Any kind of berry, mangos, papayas, kiwi fruit, et cetera make a great smoothie. Experiment with your favorites!"
Serving: *10 m |* ***Total Time:*** *10 m*

Ingredients
- 1 quart strawberries, hulled
- 1 banana, broken into chunks
- 2 peaches
- 1 cup orange-peach-mango juice
- 2 cups ice
- Add all ingredients to list

Directions
1. In a blender, combine strawberries, banana and peaches. Blend until fruit is pureed. Blend in the juice. Add ice and blend to desired consistency. Pour into glasses and serve.

Nutritional Information
- Calories: 118 kcal 6%
- Fat: 0.6 g < 1%
- Carbs: 28.5g 9%
- Protein: 1.6 g 3%
- Cholesterol: 0 mg 0%
- Sodium: 16 mg < 1%

Basil Strawberry Mango Smoothie

"This smoothie makes for a great not too sweet cool summer beverage."
Serving: *5 m |* ***Total Time:*** *5 m*

Ingredients
- 4 leaves basil
- 1 cup frozen mango pieces
- 5 hulled strawberries

- 1 cup water
- 1/4 cup white sugar, or to taste
- 3 cubes ice
- Add all ingredients to list

Directions
1. Blend the basil, mango, strawberries, and water in a blender. Add sugar and ice cubes; blend again until smooth.

Nutritional Information
- Calories: 330 kcal 17%
- Fat: 0.7 g 1%
- Carbs: 85g 27%
- Protein: 1.5 g 3%
- Cholesterol: 0 mg 0%
- Sodium: 13 mg < 1%

BFF Smoothie

"This recipe just came to me when I was looking for something healthy that my little guy would eat or drink because he eats so little. This is what I had on hand and it worked."
Serving: 10 m | Total Time: 10 m

Ingredients
- 1 cup frozen strawberries
- 1 cup plain Greek yogurt
- 1 cup frozen mango chunks
- 1/2 cup 1% milk
- 1 scoop vanilla whey protein powder
- 5 fresh mint leaves, or more to taste
- Add all ingredients to list

Directions
1. Blend strawberries, Greek yogurt, mango, milk, and protein powder together until smooth. Add mint leaves and pulse until leaves are chopped, 4 to 5 pulses.

Nutritional Information
- Calories: 335 kcal 17%
- Fat: 11.6 g 18%
- Carbs: 33g 11%
- Protein: 27.7 g 55%
- Cholesterol: 32 mg 11%
- Sodium: 202 mg 8%

Blueberry Mango Smoothie

Ingredients
- 1 tablespoon chia seeds
- 1 (6 ounce) container vanilla yogurt
- 1/2 cup mango juice
- 1/4 cup fresh blueberries
- 1/4 cup fresh mango chunks
- 1/2 teaspoon vanilla extract
- Add all ingredients to list

Directions
1. Grind chia seeds in a food processor until pulverized; add yogurt, mango juice, blueberries, mango, and vanilla extract and blend until smooth.

Nutritional Information
- Calories: 271 kcal 14%
- Fat: 2.5 g 4%
- Carbs: 54.9g 18%
- Protein: 9.1 g 18%
- Cholesterol: 8 mg 3%
- Sodium: 117 mg 5%

Coconut Banango Smoothie

"A tropical smoothie created for my daughter's school project about Florida's natural resources."
Serving: 10 m | Total Time: 10 m

Ingredients

- 1 mango - peeled, seeded, and chopped
- 1 1/2 frozen bananas, sliced
- 1/2 cup coconut milk
- 1/2 cup cold water
- 4 cubes ice, or as needed
- 1 tablespoon white sugar
- 1 teaspoon coconut extract
- 1/2 teaspoon lime zest
- Add all ingredients to list

Directions

1. Blend mango, bananas, coconut milk, water, ice, sugar, coconut extract, and lime zest in a blender until smooth.

Nutritional Information

- Calories: 268 kcal 13%
- Fat: 12.5 g 19%
- Carbs: 40.9g 13%
- Protein: 2.5 g 5%
- Cholesterol: 0 mg 0%
- Sodium: 13 mg < 1%

Creamy Mango Smoothie

"If you like mangos, you must try this luscious and creamy smoothie. It is both light and filling. You can use fresh or frozen mango chunks. There's no better way to get some calcium and fruit in for the day! Enjoy!!! If you love other fruit, add bananas, raspberries, or strawberries, if you wish."
Serving: *5 m* | **Total Time:** *5 m*

Ingredients

- 3/4 cup cold milk
- 1/4 cup vanilla yogurt
- 3/4 teaspoon vanilla extract
- 1 1/2 cups chopped fresh mango
- 3 ice cubes
- Add all ingredients to list

Directions

1.   Blend the milk, yogurt, vanilla extract, mango, and ice cubes in a blender until smooth and creamy.

Nutritional Information

- Calories: 157 kcal 8%
- Fat: 2.5 g 4%
- Carbs: 29.8g 10%
- Protein: 5.2 g 10%
- Cholesterol: 9 mg 3%
- Sodium: 61 mg 2%

Delicious Green Juice

"An easy, delicious green juice. You can substitute kale for spinach."
Serving: *5 m |* **Total Time:** *5 m*

Ingredients

- 1 cup coconut milk
- 1 banana
- 1 mango - peeled, seeded, and chopped
- 3/4 cup fresh spinach, or to taste
- Add all ingredients to list

Directions

1.   Blend coconut milk, banana, mango, and spinach together in a blender until smooth.

Nutritional Information

- Calories: 690 kcal 34%
- Fat: 49.2 g 76%
- Carbs: 69.3g 22%
- Protein: 7.6 g 15%
- Cholesterol: 0 mg 0%
- Sodium: 52 mg 2%

Easy Mango Banana Smoothie

"As a babysitter, I always look for quick, easy, healthy, and delicious recipes. Here is a great one!"
Serving: *10 m |* **Total Time:** *10 m*

Ingredients
- 2 mangos - peeled, seeded, and sliced
- 2 bananas
- 2 cups vanilla yogurt
- 2 cups milk
- Add all ingredients to list

Directions
1. Blend mangos, banana, vanilla yogurt, and milk in a blender until smooth.

Nutritional Information
- Calories: 133 kcal 7%
- Fat: 2.2 g 3%
- Carbs: 24.4g 8%
- Protein: 5.5 g 11%
- Cholesterol: 8 mg 3%
- Sodium: 66 mg 3%

Easy Mango Lassi

"This delicious and healthy shake can conquer any sweet tooth without guilt. Great for extinguishing the fire in your mouth after eating hot curries! Use Indian mangoes, preferably Alphonso or another sweet Indian cultivar. These are the orange ones, not the red and green South American variety. "
Serving: *1 h 10 m |* **Total Time:** *1 h 10 m*

Ingredients
- 2 cups plain whole milk yogurt
- 1 cup milk
- 3 mangoes - peeled, seeded, and chopped
- 4 teaspoons white sugar, or to taste
- 1/8 teaspoon ground cardamom

- Add all ingredients to list

Directions
1. Place the yogurt, milk, mangoes, white sugar, and cardamom into the jar of a blender and blend until smooth, about 2 minutes. Chill in the refrigerator for 1 hour or until cold, and serve sprinkled with a little ground cardamom.

Nutritional Information
- Calories: 195 kcal 10%
- Fat: 5.5 g 8%
- Carbs: 31.9g 10%
- Protein: 6.8 g 14%
- Cholesterol: 21 mg 7%
- Sodium: 84 mg 3%

Gloomy Day Smoothie

"This smoothie is so bright, cheerful, and delicious, it is like a blast of sunshine on even the most rainy, windy days!"
Serving: *10 m* | **Total Time:** *10 m*

Ingredients
- 1 mango - peeled, seeded, and cut into chunks
- 1 banana, peeled and chopped
- 1 cup orange juice
- 1 cup vanilla nonfat yogurt
- Add all ingredients to list

Directions
1. Place mango, banana, orange juice, and yogurt in a blender. Blend until smooth. Serve in clear glasses, and drink with a bendy straw!

Nutritional Information
- Calories: 151 kcal 8%
- Fat: 0.5 g < 1%
- Carbs: 34.6g 11%
- Protein: 4.2 g 8%
- Cholesterol: < 1 mg < 1%
- Sodium: 44 mg 2%

Honey Mango Smoothie

"This refreshing and simple drink is suitable for everyone in your family. It is a bright and sweet way to start the day."
Serving: *10 m* | **Total Time:** *10 m*

Ingredients
- 1 mango - peeled, seeded, and cubed
- 1 tablespoon white sugar
- 2 tablespoons honey
- 1 cup nonfat milk
- 1 teaspoon lemon juice
- 1 cup ice cubes
- Add all ingredients to list

Directions
1. Place the mango, sugar, and honey in a blender pitcher; pour in the milk and lemon juice, and blend until smooth. Divide the ice cubes between two serving glasses. Pour the mango smoothie over ice to serve.

Nutritional Information
- Calories: 198 kcal 10%
- Fat: 0.4 g < 1%
- Carbs: 47.5g 15%
- Protein: 4.7 g 9%
- Cholesterol: 2 mg < 1%
- Sodium: 58 mg 2%

Hong Kong Mango Drink

"A refreshing mango drink with a twist to it."
Serving: *10 m* | **Total Time:** *10 m*

Ingredients
- 1/2 cup small pearl tapioca
- 1 mango - peeled, seeded and diced
- 14 ice cubes

- 1/2 cup coconut milk
- Add all ingredients to list

Directions
1. Fill a pot with water and bring to a rolling boil over high heat. Once the water is boiling, stir in the tapioca pearls, and return to a boil. Cook the tapioca pearls uncovered, stirring occasionally, about 10 minutes. Cover and remove from heat, allowing pearls to rest for 30 minutes. Drain well in a colander set in the sink, then cover and refrigerate.
2. Place mango and ice in a blender and blend until smooth. Divide chilled tapioca pearls in 2 tall glasses, then layer the mango mixture over and top each glass with a 1/4 cup of coconut milk.

Nutritional Information
- Calories: 315 kcal 16%
- Fat: 12.3 g 19%
- Carbs: 52.9g 17%
- Protein: 1.7 g 3%
- Cholesterol: 0 mg 0%
- Sodium: 14 mg < 1%

Jalapeno Green Smoothie

"Spice up your morning by adding jalapeno pepper to your green smoothie for a refreshing on-the-go breakfast."
Serving: *5 m |* **Total Time:** *5 m*

Ingredients
- 2 bananas, broken into chunks
- 2 cups baby spinach
- 1 cup frozen mango chunks
- 1/2 teaspoon chopped jalapeno pepper, or to taste
- 1 cup water, or as desired
- Add all ingredients to list

Directions
1. Layer banana, spinach, mango, and jalapeno pepper in a blender; add water and blend until smooth, adding more water for a thinner smoothie.

Nutritional Information
- Calories: 166 kcal 8%
- Fat: 0.7 g 1%
- Carbs: 42.1g 14%
- Protein: 2.6 g 5%
- Cholesterol: 0 mg 0%
- Sodium: 30 mg 1%

Kiwi Sensation

"This is a green smoothie that I created for the September challenge of BlackWomenLosingWeight.com. Makes about 16 ounces! Prep time depends on whether the mango and kiwi are already peeled and sliced."
***Serving:** 10 m | **Total Time:** 10 m*

Ingredients
- 1 kiwi, peeled and sliced
- 1/2 cup pineapple chunks
- 1/2 cup green grapes
- 1/4 mango - peeled, seeded, and diced
- 1/4 cup water
- 1/2 cup spinach
- 2 cubes ice cubes, or as needed
- Add all ingredients to list

Directions
1. Blend kiwi, pineapple, grapes, mango, and water in a blender until smooth. Add spinach and blend again until spinach is completely integrated. Add ice and blend until ice is completely integrated.

Nutritional Information
- Calories: 102 kcal 5%
- Fat: 0.6 g < 1%
- Carbs: 25.8g 8%
- Protein: 1.3 g 3%
- Cholesterol: 0 mg 0%
- Sodium: 10 mg < 1%

Lela's Protein Mango Smoothie

"Whip up a refreshing protein vanilla mango shake."
Serving: *10 m* | **Total Time:** *10 m*

Ingredients

- 1/2 mango, chopped, or more to taste
- 1/2 cup low-fat vanilla yogurt
- 1/2 cup almond milk
- 1/2 cup ice
- 1 scoop vanilla whey protein powder
- 1 teaspoon honey, or to taste (optional)
- Add all ingredients to list

Directions

1. Blend mango, yogurt, almond milk, ice, protein powder, and honey together in a blender until smooth.

Nutritional Information

- Calories: 401 kcal 20%
- Fat: 4.4 g 7%
- Carbs: 48.7g 16%
- Protein: 44.6 g 89%
- Cholesterol: 19 mg 6%
- Sodium: 379 mg 15%

Licuado de Mango

"Every town in Mexico has someone selling this fabulously refreshing drink. Try experimenting with other fruit!"
Serving: *10 m* | **Total Time:** *10 m*

Ingredients

- 1 mango - peeled, seeded and diced
- 1 1/2 cups milk
- 3 tablespoons honey
- 1 cup ice cubes
- Add all ingredients to list

Directions

1. Place the mango, milk, honey and ice cubes into a blender. Cover and blend until smooth. Serve immediately.

Nutritional Information

- Calories: 255 kcal 13%
- Fat: 3.9 g 6%
- Carbs: 52.1g 17%
- Protein: 6.7 g 13%
- Cholesterol: 15 mg 5%
- Sodium: 82 mg 3%

Mango Banana Smoothie

"I love mangoes and fresh fruit. This is awesome to make and pack to have with you around town in a bottle, or just have for breakfast anytime."
Serving: *5 m* | **Total Time:** *5 m*

Ingredients

- 1 banana
- 1/2 cup frozen mango pieces
- 1/3 cup plain yogurt
- 1/2 cup orange-mango juice blend
- Add all ingredients to list

Directions

1. Combine the banana, mango, yogurt, and juice in a blender; blend until nearly smooth.

Nutritional Information

- Calories: 135 kcal 7%
- Fat: 0.9 g 1%
- Carbs: 30.4g 10%
- Protein: 3.2 g 6%
- Cholesterol: 2 mg < 1%
- Sodium: 39 mg 2%

Mango Cherry Smoothie

"This exotic summer fruit smoothie is a tangy, cherry-chunked, fun snack that will cool you down in the summertime."
Serving: *10 m |* **Total Time:** *10 m*

Ingredients
* 2 cups pitted cherries
* 1 cup chopped mango
* 1 cup water
* 1 cup ice cubes
* Add all ingredients to list

Directions
1. Blend cherries, mango, water, and ice cubes together in a blender until smooth.

Nutritional Information
* Calories: 158 kcal 8%
* Fat: 1.6 g 2%
* Carbs: 38g 12%
* Protein: 2.2 g 4%
* Cholesterol: 0 mg 0%
* Sodium: 9 mg < 1%

Mango Craze Juice Blend

"A great smoothie for the true mango lover!"
Serving: *5 m |* **Total Time:** *5 m*

Ingredients
* 3 cups diced mango
* 1 1/2 cups chopped fresh or frozen peaches
* 1/4 cup chopped orange segments
* 1/4 cup chopped and pitted nectarine
* 1/2 cup orange juice
* 2 cups ice
* Add all ingredients to list

Directions

1.   Place mango, peaches, orange, nectarine, orange juice, and ice into a blender. Blend for 1 minute, or until smooth.

Nutritional Information

- Calories: 150 kcal 7%
- Fat: 0.6 g < 1%
- Carbs: 38.4g 12%
- Protein: 1.3 g 3%
- Cholesterol: 0 mg 0%
- Sodium: 9 mg < 1%

Mango Lassi Come Home

"This drink is a refreshing accompaniment for your favorite curry dish."
Serving: *5 m |* **Total Time:** *5 m*

Ingredients

- 2 cups lemon-flavored yogurt
- 1 cup vanilla yogurt
- 1/4 cup milk
- 2 cups pureed mango
- 3 tablespoons honey
- 1 (12.5 fl oz) can mango nectar
- 1/8 teaspoon ground cardamom
- Add all ingredients to list

Directions

1.   Blend the lemon yogurt, vanilla yogurt, milk, pureed mango, honey, mango nectar, and cardamom together in a blender until completely combined. Serve immediately.

Nutritional Information

- Calories: 207 kcal 10%
- Fat: 3.1 g 5%
- Carbs: 41.6g 13%
- Protein: 5.9 g 12%
- Cholesterol: 9 mg 3%
- Sodium: 75 mg 3%

Mango Lassi I

"A cooling drink made with mango and yogurt, Eastern Indian Lassi."
Serving: *7 m* | **Total Time:** *7 m*

Ingredients

- 1 cup plain yogurt
- 1 mango - peeled, seeded, and chopped
- 1 tablespoon white sugar
- 3 cups cold water
- 1 pinch salt
- 4 sprigs fresh mint, garnish
- Add all ingredients to list

Directions

1. In a blender, combine yogurt, mango, sugar, water and salt. Blend until smooth. Pour into glasses and serve garnished with a sprig of mint.

Nutritional Information

- Calories: 85 kcal 4%
- Fat: 1.1 g 2%
- Carbs: 16.4g 5%
- Protein: 3.6 g 7%
- Cholesterol: 4 mg 1%
- Sodium: 44 mg 2%

Mango Lassi II

"An Indian yogurt drink - smooth, creamy, and absolutely heavenly!"
Serving: *5 m* | **Total Time:** *5 m*

Ingredients

- 2 mangos - peeled, seeded and diced
- 2 cups plain yogurt
- 1/2 cup white sugar
- 1 cup ice

- Add all ingredients to list

Directions

1. In a blender, combine mangos, yogurt, sugar and ice. Blend until smooth. Pour into glasses and serve.

Nutritional Information

- Calories: 482 kcal 24%
- Fat: 4.4 g 7%
- Carbs: 102.4g 33%
- Protein: 13.9 g 28%
- Cholesterol: 15 mg 5%
- Sodium: 179 mg 7%

Mango Lime Smoothie

"This is a delicious and refreshing summer drink. It also makes an excellent cocktail with the addition of rum. Serve in margarita glasses for a festive touch."
Serving: 10 m | Total Time: 10 m

Ingredients

- 3 mangoes, peeled, pitted, and cut into 1-inch chunks
- 2 tablespoons fresh lime juice
- 2 tablespoons confectioners' sugar
- 1 tray ice cubes
- Add all ingredients to list

Directions

1. Place the mangoes, lime juice, confectioners' sugar, and ice cubes in a blender. Blend until slushy.

Nutritional Information

- Calories: 117 kcal 6%
- Fat: 0.4 g < 1%
- Carbs: 30.7g 10%
- Protein: 0.8 g 2%
- Cholesterol: 0 mg 0%
- Sodium: 6 mg < 1%

Mango Mint Lassi with Indian Sweet Spices

"It's a great take on the famous Mango Lassi that you tend to see at various Indian restaurants because it takes the flavor to a higher and much more complex level."
Serving: *15 m* | **Total Time:** *15 m*

Ingredients
- 1 large mango - peeled, seeded, and diced
- 3 tablespoons brown sugar
- 2 tablespoons chopped fresh mint
- 1 teaspoon freshly ground star anise
- 1 teaspoon freshly ground cardamom
- 1 tablespoon lime juice
- 2 cups plain yogurt
- 3 sprigs fresh mint for garnish
- Add all ingredients to list

Directions
1. Blend the mango, brown sugar, chopped mint, star anise, cardamom, lime juice, and yogurt in a blender on high speed until smooth. Pour into glasses and garnish with fresh mint sprigs to serve.

Nutritional Information
- Calories: 228 kcal 11%
- Fat: 3 g 5%
- Carbs: 43.6g 14%
- Protein: 9.4 g 19%
- Cholesterol: 10 mg 3%
- Sodium: 121 mg 5%

Mango Oatmeal Breakfast Smoothie

"A great way to start off your day! For a creamier taste, use milk in place of orange juice. You can use vanilla yogurt instead of plain yogurt, if desired."
Serving: *10 m* | **Total Time:** *10 m*

Ingredients
- 1/2 cup orange juice
- 1/2 cup frozen mango chunks

- 1/2 banana, cut into chunks
- 1/3 cup plain yogurt
- 1/4 cup oats
- Add all ingredients to list

Directions

1. Blend orange juice, mango, banana, yogurt, and oats together in a blender until smooth.

Nutritional Information

- Calories: 290 kcal 15%
- Fat: 3.3 g 5%
- Carbs: 59.9g 19%
- Protein: 8.9 g 18%
- Cholesterol: 5 mg 2%
- Sodium: 62 mg 2%

Mango Peach Banana Smoothie

"This smoothie is absolutely incredible. My whole family loves it, young or old. Sooooooooo refreshing!"
***Serving:** 10 m | **Total Time:** 10 m*

Ingredients

- 1 (16 ounce) can mango nectar
- 1 cup peach yogurt
- 1 cup vanilla frozen yogurt
- 1 1/2 cups frozen peach slices
- 1 frozen banana, cut into chunks
- Add all ingredients to list

Directions

1. Combine mango nectar, peach yogurt, and frozen yogurt in pitcher of a blender; add peach slices and banana chunks. Blend until smooth, 30 seconds to 1 minute.

Nutritional Information

- Calories: 322 kcal 16%
- Fat: 1 g 2%

- Carbs: 74.8g 24%
- Protein: 6.9 g 14%
- Cholesterol: 6 mg 2%
- Sodium: 72 mg 3%

Mango Peach Smoothie

"You can use fresh or frozen fruit in this yummy smoothie. It tastes better if the fruit is frozen, so I freeze fresh fruit for this."
***Serving:** 10 m | **Total Time:** 10 m*

Ingredients
- 1 peach, sliced
- 1 mango, peeled and diced
- 1/2 cup vanilla soy milk
- 1/2 cup orange juice, or as needed
- Add all ingredients to list

Directions
1. Place the peach, mango, soy milk, and orange juice into a blender. Cover, and puree until smooth. Pour into glasses to serve.

Nutritional Information
- Calories: 105 kcal 5%
- Fat: 1.3 g 2%
- Carbs: 22.3g 7%
- Protein: 2.5 g 5%
- Cholesterol: 0 mg 0%
- Sodium: 29 mg 1%

Mango Pina Colada Smoothie

"This is my take on a alcohol-free pina colada."
***Serving:** 10 m | **Total Time:** 10 m*

Ingredients
- 1 mango - peeled, seeded and cubed
- 1 1/4 cups ice cubes

- 2 tablespoons white sugar
- 1 1/4 cups pineapple juice
- 1/2 cup heavy cream
- 1 (14 ounce) can coconut milk
- Add all ingredients to list

Directions

1. Place the mango cubes, ice, sugar, pineapple juice, cream, and coconut milk into a blender. Puree until smooth, pour into glasses and serve.

Nutritional Information

- Calories: 395 kcal 20%
- Fat: 32.1 g 49%
- Carbs: 28.7g 9%
- Protein: 3.1 g 6%
- Cholesterol: 41 mg 14%
- Sodium: 29 mg 1%

Mango Pineapple Green Smoothie

"A yummy, healthy smoothie made with mangoes, pineapple, banana, and spinach (shhhh!) that's sure to be a hit!"
***Serving:** 10 m | **Total Time:** 10 m*

Ingredients

- 2/3 cup frozen pineapple chunks
- 1 cup frozen mango chunks
- 1 ripe banana, sliced
- 2/3 cup fresh spinach
- 1/3 cup orange juice
- 1 cup ice
- Add all ingredients to list

Directions

1. Place pineapple, mango, banana, spinach, orange juice, and ice, respectively, in a blender and blend until smooth.

Nutritional Information

- Calories: 197 kcal 10%

- Fat: 0.6 g < 1%
- Carbs: 50.3g 16%
- Protein: 2 g 4%
- Cholesterol: 0 mg 0%
- Sodium: 16 mg < 1%

Mango Pineapple Smoothie

"I invented this one day when I had leftover mango and pineapple juice. A spoonful of cream of coconut added the sweetness and special flavor with a tropical flare. You may use frozen pineapple juice ice cubes instead for more of a slush drink (about 8 pineapple ice cubes). Enjoy!"
Serving: *10 m* | **Total Time:** *10 m*

Ingredients
- 1 cup vanilla yogurt
- 1 cup unsweetened pineapple juice
- 1/2 banana, sliced
- 1 mango - peeled, seeded, and chopped
- 1/2 cup nonfat milk
- 2 tablespoons cream of coconut
- Add all ingredients to list

Directions
1. In a blender, blend the vanilla yogurt, pineapple juice, banana, mango, milk, and cream of coconut until smooth.

Nutritional Information
- Calories: 178 kcal 9%
- Fat: 2.7 g 4%
- Carbs: 35.7g 12%
- Protein: 4.7 g 9%
- Cholesterol: 4 mg 1%
- Sodium: 61 mg 2%

Mango Watermelon Smoothie

"This is a recipe that my sister and I made, and we want to share it! Enjoy!"
***Serving:** 10 m | **Total Time:** 10 m*

Ingredients
- 5 cups cubed seeded watermelon
- 1 mango - peeled, seeded, and diced
- 1/2 cup water
- 1 tablespoon white sugar
- ice cubes (optional)
- Add all ingredients to list

Directions
1. Blend watermelon, mango, water, and sugar together in a blender until smooth.
2. Place ice into glasses and pour smoothie over ice.

Nutritional Information
- Calories: 103 kcal 5%
- Fat: 0.4 g < 1%
- Carbs: 26.3g 8%
- Protein: 1.4 g 3%
- Cholesterol: 0 mg 0%
- Sodium: 4 mg < 1%

Pawpaw Papaya And Mango Punch

"A smoothie relaxing punch."
***Serving:** 10 m | **Total Time:** 10 m*

Ingredients
- 1 cup sliced mango
- 1 cup diced, peeled papaya
- 1 cup orange juice
- 1/4 cup lime juice
- 1/4 cup white sugar, or to taste
- 1 teaspoon grated orange zest
- 4 cups water

- Add all ingredients to list

Directions

1. Place the mango and papaya into a blender. Cover, and puree until smooth; add the orange juice, lime juice, sugar, orange zest, and water. Blend well. Serve over crushed ice.

Nutritional Information

- Calories: 61 kcal 3%
- Fat: 0.1 g < 1%
- Carbs: 15.4g 5%
- Protein: 0.5 g < 1%
- Cholesterol: 0 mg 0%
- Sodium: 5 mg < 1%

Peanut Butter Mango Smoothie

Ingredients

- 1 cup vanilla yogurt
- 1 banana, broken into chunks
- 1/2 cup frozen mango chunks
- 2 tablespoons peanut butter, or to taste
- Add all ingredients to list

Directions

1. Blend yogurt, banana, mango, and peanut butter together in a blender until smooth.

Nutritional Information

- Calories: 279 kcal 14%
- Fat: 10 g 15%
- Carbs: 40.6g 13%
- Protein: 11 g 22%
- Cholesterol: 6 mg 2%
- Sodium: 157 mg 6%

Pina Colada Smoothie

"This recipe is a great on-the-go breakfast for a yummy summer morning. Or, if you are tired of snow and want a taste of summer, it is great for that, too. Super easy and it is kid-friendly! For thicker smoothie, add less milk."
Serving: *10 m* | **Total Time:** *10 m*

Ingredients
- 1 cup frozen pineapple chunks
- 1 cup frozen mango chunks
- 1 cup toasted coconut vanilla yogurt
- 1/4 cup milk
- Add all ingredients to list

Directions
1. Blend pineapple, mango, yogurt, and milk together in a blender until smooth and creamy.

Nutritional Information
- Calories: 254 kcal 13%
- Fat: 5.4 g 8%
- Carbs: 54.6g 18%
- Protein: 1.9 g 4%
- Cholesterol: 2 mg < 1%
- Sodium: 22 mg < 1%

Pink Flamingo Yogurt Smoothie

"The name says it all: slightly tropical with a combination of sweet strawberries and luscious mango. The result is as pink as a flamingo. It is a great way to start the day or delicious as a afternoon snack."
Serving: *10 m* | **Total Time:** *10 m*

Ingredients
- 10 ounces fresh strawberries, hulled and halved
- 1 cup diced mango, or more to taste
- 1 cup plain low-fat yogurt
- 1/2 cup milk
- 1/4 cup honey

- 8 ice cubes
- 4 fresh strawberries
- Add all ingredients to list

Directions

1. Put strawberries and mango in a blender; add yogurt, milk, honey, and ice cubes. Blend on high until smooth and thick. Pour smoothie into 4 glasses and garnish each with a fresh strawberry.

Nutritional Information

- Calories: 171 kcal 9%
- Fat: 1.9 g 3%
- Carbs: 36.5g 12%
- Protein: 5 g 10%
- Cholesterol: 6 mg 2%
- Sodium: 59 mg 2%

Raw Mango Monster Smoothie

Ingredients

- 1 tablespoon flax seeds
- 2 tablespoons pepitas (raw pumpkin seeds)
- 1 ripe mango, cubed
- 1 frozen banana, quartered
- 1/3 cup water, or more to taste
- 3 ice cubes
- 2 leaves kale, or more to taste
- Add all ingredients to list

Directions

1. Blend flax seeds in a blender until finely ground; add pepitas and blend until ground, about 1 minute.
2. Place mango, banana, water, ice cubes, and kale in the blender; blend until smooth, kale is fully incorporated, and the smoothie is uniform in color, about 3 minutes. Thin with more water to reach desired consistency.

Nutritional Information

- Calories: 381 kcal 19%
- Fat: 14.1 g 22%
- Carbs: 63g 20%

- Protein: 9.8 g 20%
- Cholesterol: 0 mg 0%
- Sodium: 32 mg 1%

Strawberry Mango Super Smoothie

Ingredients
- 1 1/3 cups coconut milk
- 1/2 cup aloe vera juice
- 1 tablespoon almond butter
- 1 tablespoon honey
- 2 cups frozen strawberries
- 1/2 cup frozen mango chunks
- Add all ingredients to list

Directions
1. Blend coconut milk, aloe vera juice, almond butter, and honey together in a blender until smooth; add strawberries and mango and blend on high until smooth.

Nutritional Information
- Calories: 191 kcal 10%
- Fat: 15 g 23%
- Carbs: 15.3g 5%
- Protein: 2.4 g 5%
- Cholesterol: 0 mg 0%
- Sodium: 30 mg 1%

Sugar Free Cardamom Mango Smoothie

"This Indian-inspired smoothie is creamy like a milkshake, sweet, smooth, and doesn't use sugar! It's great as a snack, and is the perfect compliment to all of my favorite Indian recipes."
***Serving:** 10 m | **Total Time:** 10 m*

Ingredients
- 2 ripe mangoes, peeled, pitted, and diced
- 1 cup fat-free plain yogurt

- 8 cubes ice
- 2/3 cup nonfat milk
- 1/4 teaspoon ground cardamom (optional)
- 1/2 cup granular sucrolose sweetener (such as Splenda®), or to taste
- Add all ingredients to list

Directions

1. Place mango, yogurt, ice, and milk into a blender. Sprinkle in cardamom and sweetener to taste. Puree until smooth, frothy, and creamy.

Nutritional Information

- Calories: 130 kcal 6%
- Fat: 0.4 g < 1%
- Carbs: 32.4g 10%
- Protein: 5.4 g 11%
- Cholesterol: 2 mg < 1%
- Sodium: 68 mg 3%

Super Healthy Fruit Smoothie

"Absolutely wonderful fruit smoothie with raspberries, blueberries, strawberries and more! I have this for breakfast every morning."
Serving: 10 m | Total Time: 10 m

Ingredients

- 1/3 cup fresh blueberries
- 1/3 cup fresh raspberries
- 4 large fresh strawberries, hulled
- 1/3 cup pomegranate juice
- 1/3 cup mango juice
- 2/3 cup milk
- 2 tablespoons honey
- Add all ingredients to list

Directions

1. Place the blueberries, raspberries, strawberries, pomegranate and mango juices, milk, and honey into a blender. Cover, and puree until smooth. Pour into glasses to serve.

Nutritional Information
- Calories: 191 kcal 10%
- Fat: 1.9 g 3%
- Carbs: 42.7g 14%
- Protein: 3.4 g 7%
- Cholesterol: 7 mg 2%
- Sodium: 37 mg 1%

Tropical Delite Smoothie

Ingredients
- 1 cup coconut milk
- 1 (15.25 ounce) can mango slices with juice
- 1/2 cup orange juice
- 1/4 cup white sugar
- 1 cup shaved ice
- 1/4 cup whipped cream, divided (optional)
- 1 tablespoon shaved milk chocolate, divided (optional)
- Add all ingredients to list

Directions
1. Place coconut milk, mango slices with their juice, orange juice, and sugar into a blender, and blend until smooth; add the shaved ice, and blend again. Pour into 4 glasses, and top each serving with a dollop of whipped cream and a sprinkling of shaved milk chocolate.

Nutritional Information
- Calories: 260 kcal 13%
- Fat: 15.9 g 24%
- Carbs: 31.5g 10%
- Protein: 1.8 g 4%
- Cholesterol: 11 mg 4%
- Sodium: 23 mg < 1%

Tropical Fruit Smoothie

"A yummy fruit smoothie made with tropical fruits."
Serving: *5 m |* **Total Time:** *5 m*

Ingredients
- 1 mango, peeled and seeded
- 1 papaya, peeled and seeded
- 1/2 cup fresh strawberries
- 1/3 cup orange juice
- 5 cubes ice
- Add all ingredients to list

Directions
1. Place the mango, papaya, strawberries, orange juice, and ice cubes in an electric blender. Process until the ingredients are smooth.

Nutritional Information
- Calories: 129 kcal 6%
- Fat: 0.6 g < 1%
- Carbs: 32.5g 10%
- Protein: 1.5 g 3%
- Cholesterol: 0 mg 0%
- Sodium: 7 mg < 1%

Tropical Sunshine Smoothie

"It is so yummy and amazingly refreshing! The color is a bright yellow so it does bring sunshine to your morning... Enjoy! For some added sweetness, agave honey is wonderful."
*Serving: 10 m | **Total Time:** 10 m*

Ingredients
- 1 banana
- 1/2 cup orange juice
- 1/2 cup cubed fresh mango
- 1/2 cup cubed fresh pineapple
- 1/2 cup coconut water
- 1/2 teaspoon freshly squeezed lime juice
- 1 sprig fresh chocolate mint, finely chopped
- Add all ingredients to list

Directions

1. Blend banana, orange juice, mango, pineapple, coconut water, lime juice, mint in a blender until smooth.

Nutritional Information

- Calories: 140 kcal 7%
- Fat: 0.6 g < 1%
- Carbs: 34.8g 11%
- Protein: 2 g 4%
- Cholesterol: 0 mg 0%
- Sodium: 66 mg 3%

Turmeric Mango Smoothie

Ingredients

- 2 banana, broken into chunks
- 1 cup frozen mango chunks
- 2 tablespoons cashew butter
- 1/8 teaspoon ground turmeric
- 2 cups water
- Add all ingredients to list

Directions

1. Combine bananas, mango, cashew butter, and turmeric powder in a blender; add water. Blend mixture until smooth.

Nutritional Information

- Calories: 253 kcal 13%
- Fat: 8.5 g 13%
- Carbs: 45.5g 15%
- Protein: 4.5 g 9%
- Cholesterol: 0 mg 0%
- Sodium: 12 mg < 1%

Ultimate Fruit Smoothie

"This is a easy but healthy smoothie that anyone can make. A little tang and a dash of sweet combine to make an excellent smoothie!"

*Serving: 10 m | **Total Time:** 10 m*

Ingredients
- 1/2 cup 2% milk
- 1/2 cup orange juice
- 1/2 mango - peeled, seeded, and cut into chunks
- 1/2 fresh peach - peeled, pitted, and sliced
- 1/4 cup fresh pineapple chunks
- 2 strawberries
- Add all ingredients to list

Directions
1. Blend milk, orange juice, mango, peach, pineapple, and strawberries together in a blender until smooth.

Nutritional Information
- Calories: 225 kcal 11%
- Fat: 3.1 g 5%
- Carbs: 46.4g 15%
- Protein: 5.8 g 12%
- Cholesterol: 10 mg 3%
- Sodium: 56 mg 2%

Vanilla Banamango Smoothie

"Trust me, it's good..."
*Serving: 15 m | **Total Time:** 15 m*

Ingredients
- 1/4 cup orange juice, or to taste
- 1 mango, sliced
- 1 frozen banana, sliced
- 2 baby carrots
- 1 (6 ounce) container vanilla yogurt
- 2 ice cubes, or as desired
- 1 teaspoon ground ginger
- Add all ingredients to list

Directions

1. Pour orange juice into the pitcher of a blender and add mango, frozen banana, carrots, vanilla yogurt, ice cubes, and ginger. Pulse several times to crush ice, then blend until smooth, 30 seconds to 1 minute.

Nutritional Information

- Calories: 192 kcal 10%
- Fat: 1.6 g 2%
- Carbs: 42.1g 14%
- Protein: 5.5 g 11%
- Cholesterol: 4 mg 1%
- Sodium: 62 mg 2%

Yummy Mango Banana Milkshake

"This mango milkshake with banana is great! Add vanilla bean ice cream if you want this to be a really rich drink. If you add too much vanilla ice cream it will start to taste like a vanilla milk shake instead of a mango drink."
Serving: *10 m* | **Total Time:** *10 m*

Ingredients

- 1/2 small mango - peeled, seeded and diced
- 1 banana, cut in chunks
- 1 scoop vanilla ice cream (optional)
- 1 tablespoon white sugar, or to taste
- 1/8 teaspoon ground cinnamon, or to taste
- 1 pinch ground nutmeg, or to taste
- 2 cups milk
- Add all ingredients to list

Directions

1. Place mango, banana, and ice cream into a blender, and sprinkle with white sugar, cinnamon, and nutmeg. Pour in milk and place the lid on the blender. Blend until smooth, then pour into cups to serve.

Nutritional Information

- Calories: 124 kcal 6%
- Fat: 3.2 g 5%
- Carbs: 20.2g 7%
- Protein: 4.6 g 9%

- Cholesterol: 12 mg 4%
- Sodium: 55 mg 2%

Chapter 7: Fruits Smoothies

***

Berry Patch Soup

Blend refrigerated leftovers with frozen banana slices to make a smoothie.
Serving: 11

Ingredients

- 3 (16-ounce) packages frozen berry mix (strawberries, raspberries, blueberries, and blackberries),thawed
- 1/2 cup honey
- 3/4 cup fat-free half-and-half
- 3 tablespoons Sauternes or other dessert white wine
- 11 tablespoons reduced-fat sour cream

Directions

1. Place one-third of berry mix in food processor or blender, and process until smooth. Strain pureed mixture through a sieve into a large bowl; discard pulp. Repeat procedure 2 times with remaining berry mix. Add honey, half-and-half, and wine to pureed mixture; stir well. Ladle soup into bowls. Dollop each with sour cream.
2. NOTE: 1 (16-ounce) package each of frozen strawberries, raspberries, and blueberries can be substituted for 3 (16-ounce) packages of frozen berry mix.

Blueberry Açaí Smoothie Bowl

Drink your morning smoothie from a bowl! With a variety of toppings, this easy breakfast movement is the healthiest way to turn a smoothie into a morning meal.
Serving: 1 | Total Time: 10 Minutes

Ingredients

SMOOTHIE
- 1 cup frozen blueberries
- 1/2 cup frozen raspberries
- 1 banana
- 1/2 cup almond milk
- 1 tablespoon honey
- 1 tablespoon açai powder

TOPPINGS
- Honey
- Sliced banana
- Granola
- Shredded toasted coconut

- Fresh raspberries

Directions
1. Combine first 6 ingredients in a blender and blend until smooth. Pour into a bowl and sprinkle with your choice of toppings.

Citrus Compote

If there are leftovers, turn them into a zesty Citrus Smoothie.
Serving: 6

Ingredients
- 2 navel oranges
- 2 blood oranges
- 2 tangerines
- 1 white grapefruit
- 1 pink grapefruit
- 1/2 cup sugar
- 2 cups gin
- Lime rind strips

Directions
1. Peel, section, and seed oranges, tangerines, and grapefruit. Cut the rind of 1 orange into thin strips. Set fruit aside.
2. Bring orange rind strips, sugar, and gin to a boil in a saucepan. Reduce heat; simmer, stirring constantly, 15 minutes or until thickened.
3. Twist lime rind strips into 6 individual compotes; layer fruit sections in compotes. Pour warm syrup over fruit.

Layered Fruit Smoothie

If island-inspired cocktails warm your soul, this layered fruit smoothie might just tip your taste buds over the edge. Pour a strawberry-banana smoothie mixture over a layer of mango smoothie for a two-tone drink that's as pretty as it is tasty.
Serving: 2

Ingredients
- 1 mango (peeled, pitted, and coarsely chopped)
- 1 1/4 cups plain low-fat yogurt
- 4 tablespoons honey

- 1 tablespoon fresh lime juice
- 1/4 teaspoon freshly grated lime zest
- 1 banana (peeled, and chopped)
- 10 medium strawberries (washed, and hulled)
- 1 tablespoon fresh lemon juice
- 1/4 teaspoon freshly grated lemon zest

Directions

1. In a blender, whirl the mango; 3/4 cup plain low-fat yogurt; 2 tablespoons honey; the fresh lime juice; 2 ice cubes; and the freshly grated lime zest until smooth. Divide mango-lime smoothie between 2 straight-sided glasses and set aside.
2. Rinse blender, then whirl the banana; the strawberries; 1/2 cup plain low-fat yogurt; 2 tablespoons honey; the fresh lemon juice; 2 ice cubes; and the freshly grated lemon zest until smooth. Layer banana-strawberry smoothie onto mango smoothie, gently spooning mixture around inside edge of each glass to create a clean horizontal line.
3. Note: Nutritional analysis is per smoothie.

Nutritional Information

- Calories 408
- Caloriesfromfat 7 %
- Protein 9.6 g
- Fat 3.3 g
- Satfat 1.7 g
- Carbohydrate 94 g
- Fiber 5.4 g
- Sodium 109 mg
- Cholesterol 8.5 mg

Mango Smoothie

Blend up this deliciously fresh and healthy mango smoothie in minutes for an icy treat.
Serving: 3

Ingredients

- 2 cups chopped mango (1 large)*
- 1/2 cup cold water
- 2 tablespoons lemon juice
- 1 (8-ounce) container vanilla yogurt

- 1/4 cup sugar

Directions

1. Process first 3 ingredients in a blender until smooth, stopping to scrape down sides. Add yogurt and sugar; process until smooth. Cover and chill 2 hours.
2. *2 cups chopped refrigerated mango slices, drained, may be substituted.

Pumped Up Smoothie

Pumped-Up Smoothie contains plenty of iron and vitamin C, giving you a smoothie that helps you stay strong.
Serving: 2

Ingredients

- 1 small banana
- 1 small orange, peeled and segmented
- 1 cup ice cubes
- 1 tablespoon raw pumpkin seeds
- 1 tablespoon agave nectar
- 2 teaspoons ground flaxseed
- 2 teaspoons hemp oil
- 1/8 teaspoon ground cloves
- Hemp seeds and additional pumpkin seeds for garnish (optional)

Directions

1. In a blender, purée first 8 ingredients (through cloves) until smooth. Pour into 2 glasses and sprinkle with pumpkin and hemp seeds, if desired; serve immediately.
2. (Recipe adapted from Thrive by Brendan Brazier)

Nutritional Information

- Calories 144
- Fat 7.8 g
- Satfat 0.9 g
- Monofat 1.7 g
- Polyfat 4.7 g
- Protein 2 g
- Carbohydrate 19 g
- Fiber 2 g
- Cholesterol 0.0 mg
- Iron 1 mg

- Sodium 2 mg
- Calcium 29 mg

Raspberry Smoothies

A fruit smoothie is also a good option for breakfast on the run.
Serving: 4

Ingredients
- 1/2 cups fresh or frozen raspberries
- 1/2 cups frozen reduced-calorie whipped topping, thawed
- (8-ounce) carton lemon low-fat yogurt

Directions
1. Combine all ingredients in a blender. Add ice cubes to reach 4-cup level. Process until smooth. Serve immediately.
2. Strawberry Smoothies: Use 1 1/2 cups sliced strawberries instead of raspberries; proceed with recipe as directed.
3. Blueberry Smoothies: Use 1 1/2 cups blueberries instead of raspberries; proceed with recipe as directed.
4. Peach Smoothies: Use 1 1/2 cups fresh or frozen sliced peaches instead of raspberries, use vanilla low-fat yogurt instead of lemon, and proceed with recipe as directed.
5. carbo rating: 28

Nutritional Information
- Calories 144
- Caloriesfromfat 0.0 %
- Fat 0.7 g
- Satfat 0.0 g
- Monofat 0.0 g
- Polyfat 0.0 g
- Protein 2.5 g
- Carbohydrate 30.8 g
- Fiber 3.1 g
- Cholesterol 0.0 mg
- Iron 0.3 mg
- Sodium 52 mg
- Calcium 107 mg

Smoothie With Benefits

No more empty calories! This pumped-up smoothie packs extra protein to keep you slim and satisfied. Now that's a Smoothie With Benefits!
Serving: 2

Ingredients
- 1/2 cup plain low-fat yogurt
- 2 cups strawberries, hulled and sliced in half
- 1/2 cup sliced banana
- 1 cup diced mango
- 2 tablespoons plain whey protein powder
- 1 tablespoon honey
- 1 cup crushed ice

Directions
1. In a blender, combine ingredients and blend until smooth. Pour into 2 large glasses.

Nutritional Information
- Calories 257
- Fat 3 g
- Satfat 1.4 g
- Monofat 0.5 g
- Polyfat 0.3 g
- Protein 16 g
- Carbohydrate 0.0 g
- Fiber 5 g
- Cholesterol 32 mg
- Iron 1 mg
- Sodium 72 mg
- Calcium 147 mg

Spiced Banana Almond Smoothie

Thanks to almond milk and almond butter, you get a double dose of the good stuff in Spiced Banana-Almond Smoothie. This smoothie satisfies as a breakfast or snack beverage.
Serving: 1

Ingredients

- 1 ripe banana
- 1 cup unsweetened almond milk
- 1 tablespoon almond butter
- 1/2 teaspoon ground cardamom
- 1 tablespoon honey
- 2 ice cubes

Directions

1.

Nutritional Information

- Calories 310
- Fat 12.3 g
- Satfat 0.8 g
- Monofat 5.2 g
- Polyfat 2.3 g
- Protein 6 g
- Carbohydrate 50 g
- Fiber 6 g
- Cholesterol 0.0 mg
- Iron 1 mg
- Sodium 217 mg
- Calcium 267 mg

Strawberry Kiwi Smoothie

This strawberry-kiwi smoothie is a great summer breakfast or pick-me-up snack. For more recipes like this, see our complete smoothie recipe collection.
Serving: 4

Ingredients

- 1 cup frozen unsweetened whole strawberries
- 1 cup low-fat vanilla soy milk
- 2 teaspoons honey
- 1/2 teaspoon vanilla extract
- 3 peeled kiwifruit, halved
- 3 firm bananas, peeled and halved

Directions

1.   Place all ingredients in a blender; process until smooth. Chill thoroughly.

Nutritional Information
- Calories 176
- Caloriesfromfat 7 %
- Fat 1.4 g
- Satfat 0.2 g
- Monofat 0.2 g
- Polyfat 0.4 g
- Protein 2.9 g
- Carbohydrate 42.2 g
- Fiber 3.9 g
- Cholesterol 0.0 mg
- Iron 1 mg
- Sodium 26 mg
- Calcium 57 mg

Conclusion

Thank you again for downloading this book!

I hope you enjoyed reading about my book!

Finally, if you enjoyed this book, please take the time to share your thoughts and post a review on Amazon. It'd be greatly appreciated!

Write me an honest review about the book – I truly value your opinion and thoughts and I will incorporate them into my next book, which is already underway.

Leave your review of my book here:

http://www.amazon.com/author/anniekate

Thank you!

If you have any questions, feel free to contact at contact@smallpassion.com

An Awesome Free Gift for You

Download Gift

http://www.smallpassion.com/awesome-gift

I want to say "**Thank You**" for buying my book so I've put together a few, awesome free gift for you **Tips and Techniques for Cooking like a Chef & Delicious Desserts!**

This gift is the perfect add-on this book and I know you'll love it.

So click the link to go grab it.

Read more my book here:

http://www.amazon.com/author/anniekate

http://www.smallpassion.com/my-cookbooks

Annie Kate

Founder of www.SmallPassion.com

* * *

www.ingramcontent.com/pod-product-compliance
Lightning Source LLC
Chambersburg PA
CBHW072033280526
45788CB00006B/2095